CREATING
RADIANT
HEALTH

CREATING RADIANT HEALTH

KEYS TO RELEASING
THE HEALING POWER WITHIN

Jeanie Traub N.H.C. and Frank Lucas N.H.C.

authorHOUSE®

AuthorHouse™
1663 Liberty Drive
Bloomington, IN 47403
www.authorhouse.com
Phone: 1-800-839-8640

The information provided in this book is for general educational purposes only. It is not intended to replace competent advice received from a knowledgeable health-care professional. It is not intended to take the place of medical advice and treatment from your personal physician. Readers are advised to consult their own doctor or other qualified health professional regarding the treatment of their medical problems. Neither the publisher nor the authors shall be liable or responsible for any possible consequences from any treatment, action, or application of supplements, herbs, or preparation to any person reading or following information in this book. If readers are taking prescription medications, they should consult with their physician and not take themselves off of medicines to start supplements without the proper supervision of a physician.

First published by AuthorHouse   02/23/2012

ISBN: 978-1-4670-6454-5 (sc)
ISBN: 978-1-4670-6455-2 (ebk)

Library of Congress Control Number: 2011918874

Printed in the United States of America

Any people depicted in stock imagery provided by Thinkstock are models, and such images are being used for illustrative purposes only.
Certain stock imagery © Thinkstock.

This book is printed on acid-free paper.

Contents

Special Weight Loss Section

This book is dedicated to my Lord and Savior Jesus Christ who died on the cross and took all of our sicknesses and diseases upon himself so we could live life in abundant health . . . and by His stripes we are healed. (Isaiah 53:5)

Starting at age twenty-nine, my health began to fail. These are some of the life altering health challenges I was treated for and the treatment method used, where applicable:

- Mitral valve prolapse dysautonomia/medication
- Arrhythmia/medication
- Chronic fatigue/medication
- Transient ischemic attacks (TIAs)
- Migraine variants/medication
- Neurological disorder/medication
- Chronic iron deficiency anemia/transfusions
- Hypoglycemia
- Ovarian cysts
- Cerebral vascular spasms/medication
- Epilepsy/medication
- Encephalopathy (left side sensory deficit)
- Cognitive disorder
- Memory loss
- **Terminal Cancer**—High-grade leiomyosarcoma/no treatment/ prayer and nutrition = total healing of all health challenges

The truth was, I was severely dehydrated; mineral deficient; poisoned by the chemicals in the packaged, preserved, and processed foods I was choosing; had digestive problems and parasites; and my body was terribly out of balance.

The truths and lessons contained in this book are what I learned to create radiant health. Thank you for learning how you can achieve the best for your health. I hope each and every one of you will be spared from the consequences of sickness, disease, and cancer. I care about you!

Love and blessings!
Jeanie

"I will praise You, for I am fearfully and wonderfully made;
Marvelous are Your works, and that my soul knows very well."
(Psalm 139:14)

"When people truly understand how wonderfully God has created their bodies and how sacred they are, they will begin to walk in the true health He has for us."

Jeanie Traub

Health and Healing

In our society today, we seem to be searching for the "magic" cure for our ailments, sickness, and disease. Many are sold on the idea there is a secret to healing our bodies out there, just waiting to be discovered. Nothing could be further from the truth.

For many years, I suffered with many diseases, took prescription medications, and hoped one day I would be healthy. I, like many others, was interested in health but did not know how to achieve it. My lack of knowledge almost killed me when, in May of 2000, I was diagnosed with terminal cancer and given a few months to live. My story can be read in *The Healing Gift—Defeating Cancer by Jeanie Traub*.

If we as a society want to stop the escalating health crisis, we will need to take personal responsibility. Paradigm shifts will have to be made, and we will have to do things differently. This generation of children is being greatly affected by the way we allow them to eat, and it is the first generation with a shorter expected lifespan than that of their parents. I am on a mission to help stop this epidemic and the number of premature deaths due to our declining health.

I am thankful that I am healthy and able to enjoy life, living life as it is intended to be. I hope you will take the challenge of learning how to live in God's best for your health. Remember to share this with others, and together we will make a difference!

The following information is provided by Frank Lucas N.H.C., president of NUPRO Nutraceutical Products Company. I fully endorse all the lessons and products, which I used to regain my health. Recipes are from the kitchen of Taunya Wills!

Introduction

There is so much information about health that it is easy to be overwhelmed. Books, infomercials, television, and radio feature experts dissecting real and imaginary health concerns that "every American should know about." Media advertisers bombard you with sound bites or glossy pages for prescriptive medicine and natural advances, and with smiling faces that extol near-miraculous additions to everyday food.

Is it any wonder that this torrent of minutiae has you confused?

Your challenge is to remove yourself from this quagmire of irrelevance and to come face-to-face with a warning similar to a sign you often see in antique stores: "You break it, you bought it." Your motto should be, "It is easier to stay healthy than to become healthy."

Certainly, you need to consider the possibility of the bad luck of an unforeseen accident or a particularly virulent infective agent, but if you manage the factors that you can control, it is more likely you will enjoy the benefits of being healthy.

Personally, I filter my choices through a question I ask myself before I choose to do something: will my body thank me for this later? When the answer is yes, more often than not, I know I am contributing to my well-being. And, I use supplements to fill the gap left by my choice to go ahead when the answer is no.

Declining health is not inevitable, but it is predictable.

The predictors are:

You are what you eat.

Joel Wallach, DVM, ND, a noted author, sought-out speaker, and producer of the controversial tape *Dead Doctors Don't Lie,* frequently points out, "If a visit to the super market results in bags of cans, boxes, and bags of food, you should throw away the contents and eat the packaging." The message is that processing, preserving, and enhancing the appearance and taste of these products significantly diminishes their nutritional value. Whole food, fresh, ripe, and properly prepared, is the superior choice.

Keep your body clean.

In 2006, the American Holistic Medical Association's *Guide to Holistic Health* reported: "There are an estimated 80,000 chemicals regularly in use today, with an additional 1,000 to 2,000 chemicals added to this list each year. Only 3 percent of them have been tested to determine whether they are toxic or carcinogenic.

In 1998, the United States released approximately 500 billion tons of toxic chemicals into the environment."

People shower or bathe every day to keep the outside of their bodies clean. It is the healthy thing to do. What about the inside? The "stuff" in the air we breathe, the water we drink, and the food we eat build up over time. Keeping the inside of your body as clean as the outside pays dividends.

Take responsibility.

You have the most to lose if your health is compromised. Stop expecting that someone or some magic machine, thing, or plant will fix what you have broken. It is your body that maintains your health, using the nutrients derived from the things you put in your mouth. Ask the question: will my body thank me for this later?

Do the best you can.

Stress, fast food, skipping meals, and inactivity is one set of predictors; rest, a healthy diet, and moderate exercise is another. Make changes where you can and then use supplements to fill the gap. Just remember: "You break it, you bought it."

Health is a journey that features you, the person with the most to gain—or lose—when you choose a path.

Healthy People Don't Get Sick

Sick Care Versus Health Care

Background

Today, the science of senescence, the study of how the human body ages, repeatedly shows that the human body can live well beyond today's average life span of approximately seventy-eight years. And, that the body is fully capable of achieving and maintaining the preferred state—healthy, active, and vital—during the totality of life.

As early as 1965, pioneers of senescence, like Dr. Leonard Hayflick, observed the phenomenon of programmed replacement of cells in the human body. They found that while some cells are replaced more quickly, every cell—all tissue, every organ, system, and structure in the human body—is replaced every seven years. Each cell is reproduced exactly as it was the first time using a recipe programmed at conception, called DNA.

Estimates are that the body replaces up to 300 billion cells every day to maintain the viability of 750 trillion cells that make up the human body. This mind-challenging task is accomplished by combining the nutritional components derived entirely from the diet.

The increasing costs for insurance and medical treatment, the expense and safety of prescriptive medicine, trips to the doctor's office, and diminished quality of life makes being unhealthy very expensive. The saying, "It is easier to stay healthy than recover what has been lost," is exactly right.

Analysis

Healthy is the normal state for the human body. Sick and diseased are not!

There are four situations that affect wellness in the United States.

- Bad luck at birth: if you were ever healthy, it is unlikely that genetics has anything to do with your state of health.
- Infection and/or infestation: viruses, bacteria, fungi, or parasites.
- Injury or accident.

- Degenerative disease: the gradual decline of your overall feeling of well-being.

The allopathic medical community, for the most part, addresses the first three situations of the well-being conundrum. The fourth, degenerative disease, continues to be an issue.

People should be concerned when their health begins to decline.

Many people do nothing. Whether they choose to ignore the signs of degenerative disease for financial reasons, personal beliefs, or ignorance, they accept the ravages of declining health as part of aging and elect to suffer in silence, needlessly.

Other people expect someone else to be responsible.

- Experience the elation when their medical doctor gives them a little piece of paper with the prescription for something to fix their complaint.
- Accept the bothersome and sometimes dangerous side effects.
- Make a lifelong commitment to the prescription and the side effects.
- Experience the disappointment when nothing changes or something equally or more troublesome pops up.
- Repeat the cycle over, over, and over until all of the little pieces of paper take control of their lives.
- Accept the hopelessness of more little pieces of paper and declining health.

Some people are learning that they have an alternative.

- Accept the responsibility for their own well-being.
- Recognize it is easier to invest in health than to pay for illness.
- Accept that to change the way things are, they need to change some of the things they do.
- Become confident that given the proper nutrients, care, and enough time, the body can and will repair itself.
- Make reasonable choices that help them experience the joy of health.

Three Approaches to Managing Your Health

The first approach is to *do nothing*.

This approach accepts the decline in well-being as inevitable, condemning sufferers for the remainder of their life. Frankly, not a very appealing prospect.

The second approach is to *react to a symptom.*

This approach is effective when there is a definitive cause, a beginning and an end. It involves someone asking the question, what brings you in today? Depending on your answer, you will receive a service. In the case of certain infections, injuries, or accidents, the intervention stops the decline attributable to the complaint, which provides the body the time it needs to react to the situation. "It isn't the gun shot that kills you, it is your body's inability to react to the change of circumstance," best describes this approach. Emergency room personnel stop the bleeding, stabilize the victim, and then wait for the damage to heal.

Ideally, the reactive approach should have a beginning and an end. Kill bacteria with an antibiotic; wait for the body to heal. Repair an injury; wait for the body to heal. Suture the wound; wait for the body to heal.

When the cause is less clear, the reactive approach addresses the complaint; it becomes an intervention without an end. This limitation of the reactive approach contributes to frustration and a sense of hopelessness that many people experience when they are trapped in the reactive approach.

The third approach is to *promote and maintain health proactively.*

This approach is grounded in a tenet that deficiencies in the modern diet contribute to a gradual decline in general health, the integrity of bodily structure tissues, and organs that are produced or replaced on a daily basis. Further, besides a general malaise, this shortfall in the diet negatively impacts the body's ability to respond to incidental circumstances such as infection, accidents, and injury.

The proactive approach contends that the complaints associated with dietary deficiencies can be overcome, or avoided altogether, with the judicious use of dietary supplements.

The proactive approach may be effective when used to:

- Sustain the healthy body
- When there is no satisfactory finding of a definitive cause for a particular circumstance
- When the reactive approach presents an unsatisfactory outcome

Choosing to employ the proactive approach, the individual examines past circumstances, various daily actions, and choices that may affect overall well-being, making appropriate changes to address the impediments while creating a protocol to change the unsatisfactory outcome. Many people find this approach to be hopeful because of their positive involvement in the process and the experiential outcomes. Others, unfortunately, are overwhelmed with the responsibility.

Conclusion

Sadly, the cost of insurance premiums is expanding the number of people who choose to do nothing. In the end, this will certainly exacerbate the consequences of neglect and elevate the level of profound intervention.

The medical establishment prefers that people elect to follow the status quo—accept the reactive approach as the means to address their issues of well-being. National attention, focusing on the dangers and recalls of several mainstay drugs, has the public examining the benefits of total reliance on the reactive approach to health and, frankly, questioning the wisdom of that reliance.

The sensibility of a proactive approach to well-being offers a real alternative. It provides those who cannot afford the price of admission for the reactive approach an affordable means to address well-being. Also, it offers people who have become frustrated and disenchanted, or other people who elect to take control of their own destiny, the opportunity to make a positive contribution to their well-being.

Insanity is doing the same thing over and over, expecting a different outcome. You must change the things you do to change the way things are.

Truth #1: Cleanliness Is Next to Godliness

Are You Clean Inside? Who hasn't heard the expression, "Cleanliness is next to Godliness," thousands of times?

- You have showered at least fifteen thousand times . . . so far.
- You have brushed your teeth thirty thousand times . . . so far.
- You have washed your hands on a regular basis.

Most people practice good hygiene.
It is the healthy thing to do, and it minimizes offending appearance and odors.

What about the inside?
Did you know: you have nine square feet of skin on the outside of your body and ten thousand square feet on the inside?
Consider this: could the very things that affect the cleanliness of the outside of your body affect the inside?

Have you ever thought about cleaning the inside of your body?
Probably not. Of all the different possibilities, the state of one's intestines is probably at the bottom of most people's lists. Irritable bowel syndrome, constipation, gas, diverticulitis, and colon cancer are simply not things that people think about *until it is too late*.

> Environmental toxins, an unhealthy diet,
> internal toxins, and parasites
> are threatening your health.
>
> The secret to great health can be described in
> these words:
> "Cleanse the inside of your body!"

What You Must Know About Regularity
There is an epidemic in America. People are buying laxatives and using prescription drugs and commercial fiber supplements to no avail. Constipation, gas and bloating, weight gain, fatigue, burning stomach,

skin problems, and a host of other complaints are taking the fun out of life.

The expression, "Death begins in the colon," is right on point! Sadly, the accumulating toxic wastes produce lots of suffering, while you are being slowly poisoned from the inside.

Don't believe it? "Autopsies often reveal colons that are plugged up to 80 percent with waste material" (*Vegetarian Times*, March 1998). Most people endure the complaints of irregularity when they could put an end to their suffering very simply by becoming as clean on the inside as they are outside.

What You Must Know About Pollution

We are all exposed to thousands of toxins and chemicals every day—at work, in the home, in the air we breathe, the water we drink, the food we eat. Plus, we are eating more sugar and preserved and processed foods, and taking more medicine than ever. Our bodies are being overwhelmed by trying to eliminate all of the things we inhale and ingest every day. Unfortunately, most of this debris simply accumulates in our cells, tissues, blood, and organs (such as the colon, liver, and brain), where it is stored for an indefinite length of time, causing all kinds of complaints and leading toward a decline in your quality of life and health.

What You Must Know About Parasites

Every living thing has at least one parasite that lives inside or on it, and many, including humans, have far more. In fact, the *National Geographic*, in a documentary titled *The Body Snatchers (2000),* reports, "Parasites have killed more humans than all the wars in history."

Scientists are just beginning to appreciate how powerful these hidden inhabitants can be. Their research is pointing to a remarkable possibility: parasites rule the world. They live undetected in the body, damaging tissue, robbing your body of valuable nutrients, and burdening your body with the additional wastes produced by the parasite. Like it or not, you probably have one or more parasites living in your body, living undetected until there are more of them than your body can support. At that point, you will start paying the price extracted by parasites.

What You Must Know About Food

Processing robs food of its nutritional value. The chemicals in preserved foods lead to poor digestion, causing a toxic buildup of sludge in the intestines and on the intestinal wall, including the colon. This buildup can slow digestion and block nutritional uptake. And because the sludge is waste material, they produce toxins that pour into your bloodstream and are distributed throughout the body.

The answer to the question, "Are you clean inside?" is: "Probably not!" The combination of environmental toxins, an unhealthy diet, internal toxins, and parasites poses a threat to your health.

The next question is, Will cleansing help me? The answer is a resounding yes!

How good do you feel after a nice, hot shower? How great will you feel after a good cleaning on the inside?

The environment, the food we eat and the way we live virtually guarantee that everyone needs to freshen up their body.

And feel better because they did.

Evaluate yourself.

How do you know if it is time to clean the inside of your body?	
It is time to free your body from accumulated toxins, parasites, and other waste materials if you experience one or more of the following:	
Frequent fatigue and low energy Flatulence, gas, and bloating Excess weight Food sensitivities and allergies Impaired digestion Irritability, mood swings Bad breath and foul-smelling stools Parasites in stool Frequent colds and illnesses	Recurring headaches Chronic constipation Irritable bowel syndrome (IBS) Protruding belly pooch Powerful food cravings Skin problems, rashes, etc. Metallic taste in mouth Hemorrhoids Yeast infections

A Quick Overview for Cleansing Your Body

1. *Sweep away the barriers that are dragging you down*. Cleanse the colon and digestive tract to clear away the toxic plaque, debris, and parasites. Plus, "cleaning up that mess" helps detoxify your liver, blood, and brain tissues—basically, the first step will purify your whole body.
2. *Restore and balance the intestinal tract.* Use digestive enzymes to help break down food and friendly microbes to balance digestion, support the immune system that protects you, and along with enzymes, strengthens the body and supports the elimination of wastes thoroughly and often.

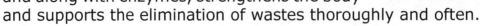

3. *Address parasites twice each year—spring and fall.*
4. *Support the body's ability to cleanse itself with diet and nutraceutical supplements.*

There are several cleansing methods, some of which can be quite harsh. Most detoxification experts feel that a one- or two-week program is simply not sufficient, especially when you consider that it took years or even decades to accumulate all the toxins in the colon and other parts of the body. A more realistic approach takes at least thirty days or even longer, depending on the level of toxicity in one's body.

The first objective of a cleansing program is to be thorough yet gentle. One effective and safe way is the Radiant Health Plan developed by NUPRO.

The two-step program (each lasting thirty days) offers you a gentle, comprehensive, thorough, all-natural detoxification program. Once you complete the cleansing and restoring programs, a third step provides a long-term plan to protect your new lease on life.

> Dr. Paul Bragg, a pioneer of natural medicine and author of dozens of successful books writes, "When the body is cleansed, it releases the toxic poisons and becomes purified . . . then there are no longer distressful toxins to cause health problems!" (Bragg Healthy Lifestyle, Vital Living to 120! P.65) The secret to great health can be described in these words:
> Cleanse the Inside of Your Body!

Truth #2: Disease Is an Abnormal Condition

Degenerative disease is:

the gradual, almost imperceptible decline in health as time passes. It is an unnatural state of health that keeps you running back and forth to the doctor for something to stop the symptoms of something for which there is no cure.

Degenerative disease is a thief that steals the quality of life as people age.

You won't wake up one morning and remark, "I've got degenerative disease! It doesn't happen that way. This thief sneaks up on you and then—wham—you've been had.

There are a few possibilities to consider: Parasites in Humans

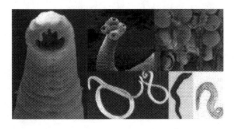

Parasites are a topic most people do not want to consider.

People believe that parasites are limited to third world countries and are uncommon in the United States.

Nothing could be further from the truth!

It has been estimated that 85 percent of the North American adult population has at least one form of parasite living in their bodies. Some authorities feel this figure may be as high as 95 percent. Valerie Saxon, N.D. in her book, Every Body Has Parasites,(p. 80), writes, ". . . that 80 to 90 percent of the American public has parasites. My own in house studies suggests 100 percent, . . ."

How can we possibly get infected in the United States?

Here are just a few of the ways: increased international business and tourist travel, armed forces returning home, immigration, contaminated water supplies, swimming in contaminated lakes and streams, and your pets or other people's pets. Food supplies—such as pork, processed meats, uncooked meats, chicken, lamb, and even fish—may contain human parasites.

Like it or not, everyone is affected by parasites.

Parasites are organisms that derive nutrition and shelter by living in or on another organism—living and dying in the host (your body). Along the way, they reproduce to assure that there are future generations to live and die in their host—producing others to be passed on to another unsuspecting host. Just about any part of your body is vulnerable to infestation: the lungs, liver, esophagus, brain, blood, muscles, joints, skin . . . and even your eyes!

	Over 150 different types of colon parasites, intestinal parasites, and organ parasites affect human well-being.
• **Tired** • **Bloated** • **Hungry** • **Allergies** • **Rashes** • **Itching**	• Parasites are not limited to third world countries or poor people. • They are found in all climates. • Besides the probability of local parasitic contamination, natural disasters, flooding, accidents at upstream treatment plants, increased mobility, international air travel, immigration, and armed forces personnel returning home significantly increase the likelihood of a parasitic contamination delivered from some other place.

The issue is not whether you have parasites, because you do!
The question is how many you have!

Parasites may do any or all of six things:

1. *Cause physical damage* to the body by perforating the intestines, circulatory system, lungs, liver, and other organs and tissue, essentially making Swiss cheese of them. Food allergies, for example,

may be an indication of a parasitic condition of the intestine, which allows food to leak into the lymph system, causing an immune response to the leaked material.

2. *Weaken, damage, or block certain organs* just with their presence.
3. *Lump together into a mass.* Parasites may exist in the brain, heart, lungs, other organs, structures, and tissue of your body.
4. *Weaken the host by robbing the host of essential nutrients*, taking a portion of the nutrients on which the host depends.
5. *Poison the host with their wastes.* In the best case, the host does double duty, disposing of its waste and that of the parasites. Worse, when the host has difficulty disposing of the parasite's wastes, a poisoning called verminous intoxication occurs.
6. *Fool the host's immune system* into believing the parasite is part of its body. The parasitic population is allowed to grow, unaffected by any of the body's normal defense mechanisms.

Symptoms of intestinal parasites, colon parasites, and organ parasites may include:

Constipation: due to worms that block the intestine.

Diarrhea: certain parasites release a hormone-like substance that can lead to a watery stool.

Gas and bloating: Some human parasites that live in the small intestine cause inflammation that produces gas and bloating.

Irritable bowel syndrome: Human parasites can irritate, inflame, and coat the lining of the intestines, causing symptoms of this disease.

Joint and muscle aches and pains: Parasites can migrate and become enclosed in a sac in joint fluids; worms can do this in muscles as well.

Anemia: Some intestinal worms attach themselves to the lining of the intestines, feeding on the vital nutrients of the host.

Allergies: Parasites can penetrate the intestinal lining and allow large, undigested food particles into the body, which can create the immune system response that is often assumed to be an allergy.

Skin conditions: Intestinal worms can cause hives, rashes, weeping eczema, and a whole host of other skin conditions.

Nervousness: Human parasites create wastes and toxic substances that can be severe irritants to the central nervous system. Restlessness or anxiety are often the symptoms associated with these parasitic wastes.

Sleep disturbances: Multiple awakenings at night between the hours of 2 and 3 AM are possibly caused by the liver's attempt to flush toxic wastes, produced by parasitic infestations, out of the body.

Tooth grinding and clenching: This has been observed in patients with known cases of human parasitic infestations.

Chronic tiredness: Parasites steal your food and nutrients and overwhelm your body with their wastes. This can cause fatigue, flulike complaints, apathy, impaired concentration, depression, and memory problems.

Immune system dysfunctions: Human parasites depress the immune system by continuously stimulating the immune system. Over time, this exhausts your defense system.

Excess weight, acne, and others: These can be telltale signs of parasitic invasion: excessive hunger, asthma, bad taste in the mouth, bad breath, epilepsy, migraines, and even heart and other degenerative diseases.

Everyone can be affected by intestinal parasites, colon parasites, and organ parasites. They rob you of essential nutrition as they live, reproduce, and die, weakening and damaging your body. They create wastes that burden or even poison your body, repeating the cycle over and over with each new generation, in increasingly larger numbers.

Nothing New
Humans have been using natural means to deal with parasites since the beginning of recorded history.

- They dealt with parasites in the spring, after a long winter of close contact with other humans,
- in the fall, after a summer of contamination from the environment, water, food, and soil, or
- anytime they felt their energy and vitality slipping away.

Classic herbal methods for managing parasites include wormwood, cloves, and black walnuts. More modern nutraceutical formulations have given rise to even more efficient natural means for dealing with parasites.

Why wait? The benefits of dealing with parasites, interrupting their life cycles, and protecting yourself from further invasion are obvious. Learn how you can deal with parasites at the end of this book.

Promote Regularity and Manage Constipation

A critical function of the human body is the elimination of waste.

The estimated time between eating a meal and elimination of solid waste is six hours. Studies show that some people are storing between 12 and 40 pounds of solid wastes due to constipation and accumulating wastes.

What is Constipation?
Constipation means that a person has three bowel movements or fewer in a week, the stool is hard and dry and sometimes it is painful to pass. You may feel "draggy" and full.

The bad news is: constipation can kill you.
The worse news is: it will make you very sick before it does.

There are professionals who are willing to tell you that regularity "depends on the person." Well, that's not true! People should have at least one bowel movement every day—preferably one after each meal. That's right—one well formed, 2" around, 6" cigar—after each meal.

When you understand what causes constipation, you can begin the process of managing constipation.

For most people, the number 1 cause of constipation is eating too many processed and fast foods, too little exercise and not drinking enough water—you can take steps to manage constipation or prevent it altogether.

The food you eat, how much you exercise and how much water you drink—everyday—is a major factor for most people. But, there are other factors, too.

What can you do to manage constipation?

Man has been using synthetic, chemical compounds
in food and for medicine for only 100 years.

Check the food you eat.
Packaged, preserved and fast food contain chemicals that preserve it for "shelf life" at the supermarket and at home, flavor it, color it, may interfere with digestion, may be putting your digestive tract to sleep or poisoning your body straight away. Cutting back on processed, packaged foods, and fast food lunches is important when you are beginning to manage

constipation. Packing a lunch from home is not very glamorous but it is a very good alternative.

Check the medicines you take.
Medicines that you take for another problem might cause constipation—ask your doctor (or search the internet) if your prescriptions might be at fault. They include pain pills, pills with codeine in them, some antacids, iron pills, diuretics (water pills), and medicines for depression. Ask your Doctor if there is an alternative prescriptive medicine to help you manage your constipation. Don't forget the over the counter medicines either. They can play a role, too.

Use OTC and prescriptive laxatives as a last resort and only under professional advice.

Laxatives (in any form) are medicines that will make you pass a stool. Your doctor may recommend laxatives for a limited time. **Be advised**: The FDA is warning consumers not to use oral sodium phosphate (OSP) bowel cleanser products because of the risk of acute kidney injury. These products are routinely used as bowel cleansers before colon examinations, other medical procedures and in OTC (over-the-counter) products for bowel cleansing.

> Man has been using herbs for food and medicine
> since the dawn of time.

Functional constipation means that the bowel is healthy but not working properly. It is often the result of poor dietary habits and lifestyle. Changing what you eat, what you drink and how much you exercise will help relieve and prevent constipation. Here are some positive steps you can take to manage your constipation:

Eat more fiber.
Fiber helps form soft, bulky stool. It is found in many fresh vegetables, fruits and whole grains. One good suggestion is "The Perfect Breakfast". The recipe can be found at the end of this book. It is easy, tastes great, gives you a terrific start in the morning, helps with cholesterol, high blood pressure and constipation. NOTE: Be sure to add fiber a little at a time, so your body gets used to it slowly.

Limit white flour foods, dairy, sugar, starches and starchy vegetables.
Foods that have little or no fiber such as ice cream, cheese, meat, snacks like chips and pizza, and processed foods such as instant mashed potatoes

or already-prepared frozen dinners have little or no fiber and can make the situation worse. One of the first questions is: What do I cook? There are 10 recipes at the end of this book that are great tasting and easy to prepare. They are a terrific way to painlessly manage constipation and eat your way to regularity.

Drink plenty of water, eat lighter meals and soups.
Liquid helps keep the stool soft and easy to pass, so it's important to drink enough fluids. The formula for water is: drink 1/2 your body weight in ounces (up to a maximum of 128 ounces) every day. NOTE: Try not to drink liquids that contain sugar, caffeine or alcohol. Caffeine and alcohol tend to dry out your digestive system.

Get more exercise.
Regular exercise helps your digestive system stay active and healthy. You don't need to become a great athlete. A 20- to 30-minute walk every day may help.

Allow yourself enough time to have a bowel movement.
Sometimes we feel so hurried that we don't pay attention to our body's needs. Make sure you don't ignore the urge to have a bowel movement, and then allow enough time for it to happen.

Choose a natural nutraceutical supplement to *promote bowel function* or a natural, *thorough whole body cleanse*, like the Radiant Health Plan at the end of the book, to sweep away the years of accumulation, restore balance and function.

These simple steps, along with a natural night cleanser, can help you manage constipation and, depending on your commitment to changing the things that are causing the problem in the first place, support regularity.

19

Truth #3: Healthy Digestion Keeps a Healthy Body

Digestion Is the Highway to Health or the Road to Ruin

- Regularity
- Diarrhea
- Constipation
- Energy
- Moods
- Obesity
- Skin
- Gas
- Belching
- Bloating
- Immunity
- Allergies
- Headache
- Heartburn
- Food Tolerance

Most people would rather not think or talk about matters of digestion. They choose to deal quietly with the consequences of neglecting this aspect of their health.

People pay a terrible price when their digestion goes wrong! When it strikes, you will consider almost anything to get relief. Unfortunately, most of the time people deal with the symptoms, not the problem.

Many people have discovered that they are far better off restoring the digestive process.

Digestion is the cornerstone of radiant health.

It is an elegant process.

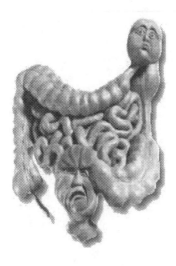

- Food is taken in
- Broken into smaller parts
- Liquefied and treated with acid
- Processed by an army of microbes until it can be absorbed
- After which, the by-products are discarded

The body doesn't benefit from the food we eat; it relies on the digested nutrients it can absorb. Digestion is an intricate dance between enzymes, stomach acids, and microbes. One partner prepares the food for the next with one goal: to provide absorbable nutrients to keep the body strong and healthy.

The digestive tract is a twisting, turning tube with pouches and valves. The functions are:

- Provide an orderly path for food to follow
- Create nutrition to sustain the body
- Separate caustic agents from delicate body structures
- Protect the body from toxic substances, infectious microorganisms, and parasites
- Gather the remnants of undigested food, toxic substances, infectious organisms, parasites, and the wastes produced by the body
- Quickly expel these toxins and wastes to avoid contaminating the body

Digestion is more complex than it may seem.
It is an intricate dance between enzymes, stomach acids, and microbes, with the goal of—creating and maintaining a strong, healthy body.

Enzymes
The digestive tract converts food into nutrition to sustain the body. The processes involved in the conversion of food to nutrition are fully dependent on the interplay of digestive enzymes, stomach acids, and microbes.

Dr. Edward Howell (*Enzyme Nutrition*, Avery Publishing, Wayne, NJ, 1985, p.33) writes: "Enzymes are substances that make life possible. They are needed for every chemical reaction that takes place in the human body." We are completely dependent on these metabolic enzymes for virtually every body function: energy, alertness, memory, thinking, and hundreds of other activities are totally dependent on enzymes.

Dr. Edward Howell identifies three types of enzymes—digestive enzymes, metabolic enzymes, and food enzymes—which exist in raw, unprocessed, uncooked food.

Enzymes, while very powerful, are fragile. Cooking and processing foods destroys the raw food enzymes. A synopsis of Dr. Howells' book is, a diet composed of cooked and processed food, in which the natural enzymes are destroyed, leads to enzymes insufficiency and stresses the organs which secrete enzymes.

"Enzymes may be damaged or excreted during the process of digestion, absorption and elimination and are not recycled. We depend on raw food enzymes to replace these damaged and lost enzymes. A lifetime of eating 'dead foods' is a contributing factor," in the decline from radiant health.

The short version is: if your diet consists of cooked, packaged, processed, and preserved foods, Dr. Howell advocates supplementing your diet with enzymes.

Probiotics

The definition of "probiotic" is "for life." It is the science of administering living, friendly microbes to promote and maintain health.

Prevailing estimates are that the intestines of one human contain more beneficial microbes than there are people on earth. Babies are born with germ-free intestines, rapidly acquiring an army of beneficial microbes from their mothers during and shortly after birth. Without this natural microbial inoculation, the newborn cannot complete digestion and will die of starvation. Once established, the relationship with this vast internal ecosystem of microbes, called intestinal flora, influences every person's physical health, mental health, and longevity.

During digestion, food is subjected to the action of enzymes, stomach acids, and gastric juices. This partially digested food (called chyme) is turned over to this army of microbes to create the nutrition that supports the body and keeps it healthy. It supports and addresses:

- Regularity
- Diarrhea
- Constipation
- Gas, bloating, and belching
- Liver function

- Vitamin uptake
- Mineral uptake
- Calcium absorption
- B vitamin production

- Cholesterol
- Immune function
- Intestinal function

Disruptions in any or all of these functions may be an indication these crucial microbes are out of balance.

Your intestinal microbes can be damaged by:

- Packaged and processed food
- Stress
- Antibiotics
- Alcohol
- Chlorinated water

- Food additives
- Food preservatives
- Constipation
- Prescriptive drugs
- OTC medications

- Birth control pills
- Hormone replacement therapy
- Pesticides
- Pollution
- X-rays

The regular use of a probiotic* supplement is one way to assure a vital population of intestinal microflora.

*Probiotics, from the Greek "for life", is the science of administering living, friendly microbes to promote and maintain the health of the digestive ecosystem.

It's Your Life—It's Your Choice!

Truth #4: Your Body Can Heal Itself

Learn Your Body's Rules

Regardless of whether you are in the glow of health, feel health slipping away, or are experiencing the affects of neglecting your body, the best news you will ever hear is, "It's not over 'til it's over!"

- The body is adaptable.
- The body is resilient.
- The body is forgiving.

The body sustains itself by using nutrition for three things:

1. Energy to perform all of the different functions involved in living
2. Replace or repair tissue that has worn out or been damaged in the process of living
3. Protect itself from infection, infestations, or profound oxidative damage

The process is straightforward:

1. You select and eat food.
2. The food is liquefied and treated with stomach acid and gastric juices resulting in chyme.
3. The chyme is digested by an army of intestinal microbes.
4. Nutrition, produced by the microbes, passes through the intestinal wall into the bloodstream and is delivered throughout the body to be used in the production of energy and cellular repair or replacement.
5. Wastes and cellular debris are passed back into the bloodstream and delivered back to the intestines, where it is combined with indigestible food and eliminated from your body. *Note:* Your body should store two meals: one being processed for nutritional value and another being prepared for elimination. When you introduce more food into the system, wastes should be eliminated to help avoid contamination from ingested toxins and organisms, debris, and waste.

Your body is composed of:

1. Water—55 to 60 percent
2. Protein—20 percent
3. Fat—15 percent
4. Minerals—5 percent
5. Carbohydrates—2 percent
6. Vitamins—<1 percent

To help you understand the scope of the tasks performed by your body, the biology of science, Senescence, suggests that:

- Your body is composed of 750 trillion cells.
- It replaces *every* cell *every* seven years.
- It builds 300 billion new cells every night.

Simply stated, your body depends on a reliable, diverse source of these nutritional components to stay healthy. If they are not readily available in sufficient amounts and in the proper ratios to accommodate your body's needs, your body begins to decline.

In a perfect world, you would provide your body everything it needs to flourish by drinking eight to ten eight-ounce glasses of water and eating five to seven servings of raw, fresh, ripe vegetables and two fruits every day. You would augment your diet with two to four ounces of muscle meat two to three times each week. Scientists and nutritionists all agree that the most healthy people eat like this. And, there is a direct relationship between the quality of your health and the quality of your diet.

Sadly, we don't live in a perfect world. Some people are unaware of the consequences of choosing to rely on a diet of processed and preserved foods. Others actually believe fast food is nutritious. Other people know better, but because of time and convenience, choose to ignore the consequences of neglecting their diet.

What Are the Options?

1. Do the best you can.
2. Drink water instead of soda, coffee, or tea.
3. If you feel hungry, drink a glass of water first. The sensations of hunger and thirst are often confused; most of you are dehydrated!
4. Reduce the amount of white foods in your diet (i.e., dairy products, white wheat flour products [white bread and pasta], processed sugar products [candy, soda, corn syrup], white rice, and fewer root starches like white potatoes.

5. Eat fresh foods whenever possible. Preservatives stop food from spoiling, but they affect digestion. A good rule of thumb is, "If the food you eat won't spoil in two or three days, you will have trouble digesting it."
6. Stop expecting there is some chemical compound, magical herb, or secret formula that will fix what you have broken.
7. Choose a supplement program and stick to it! The simple fact is supplements compensate for deficiencies in your diet. When your dietary choices create a deficiency, you should consider filling the gap with dietary supplements to provide your body the nutritional resources it needs to carry out the various functions that keep you healthy, vital, and youthful.

If you eat mostly cooked foods, add a plant based enzyme supplement like Bene•Zymes™. Containing a cross-section of plant enzymes, Bene•Zymes™ provides the food enzymes that cooking destroys. It helps support speedy digestion and provides the raw materials for the creation of the enzymes that operate your body.

If your diet consists of mostly prepared and packaged meals, add a non-dairy probiotic supplement that does not require refrigeration like Bene•Flora™. Containing a probiotic intestinal inoculant, Bene•Flora™ supports nutrition uptake by helping maintain the army of microbes affected by preservatives and other food additives.

One final thought: The natural state of your body is health.

It makes more sense to invest in maintaining your health than to pay to repair what is broken. When you experience a decline in this natural state, it is important to remember the healthiest people provide their bodies with the nutritional resources to maintain it. You, like thousands of others, may benefit from choosing to fill a nutritional deficiency with a dietary supplement to help right your ship.

*How and where to get supplements are at the end of this book.

Lesson 1

Essential, Natural Elixir

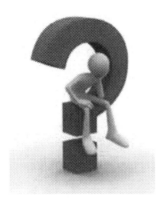

If you were shown a substance that:

- Aids weight loss
- Clears complexion
- Improves breathing
- Improves endurance

- Reduces puffiness
- Improves circulation
- Improves digestion
- Fights constipation

would you be interested?

This could be the wonder product of the century!

I'll bet you are you asking:
"How much does it cost?" and "Where can I get it?"

Here's how:
Go to your kitchen sink, fill a glass with water, and drink it. That's right—it's water!

Incredible as it may seem, water is the most important component of good health known to man.

In fact, 55 percent to 60 percent of the body's weight is water.
Water is the body's solvent: it thins blood, carries away toxins, helps metabolize fat, liquefies consumed food, rinses out organs, balances electrolytes to support nerve function, and carries hormones for endocrine function. In short, it is the body's magic potion.

However, when the body gets less water than it needs, it perceives the situation as a threat to survival and begins to conserve every drop. Many of the cleansing functions of water are affected, as it reuses and reuses and reuses the conserved, filthy water.

Drinking enough water is the best treatment for a whole litany of things:
headache, constipation, digestion, sluggishness, clarity of mind, water retention, weight gain—all symptoms of dehydration.

27

There is a good rule of thumb for drinking enough water.

Divide your body weight by two. The result is the number of ounces of water to consume every day.

Caffeinated beverages such as coffee, soda, energy drinks, and certain teas, are diuretics; they force the body to expel water. If you consume caffeinated beverages, compensate for their effect by drinking two ounces of water for each ounce of these beverages

If you are trying to lose weight or are not healthy, increase the amount by 20 percent.
Contrary to popular opinion, juices, soups, and other liquids that require digestion do not count. Water is water.

Follow this schedule to utilize water effectively:

- Morning (right after rising): consume one quart of water during a thirty-minute period.
- Noon: consume one quart of water during a thirty-minute period.
- Evening: consume one quart of water during a thirty-minute period.
- Drink the remainder of your requirement throughout the day.

The body's signal for hunger and thirst are similar and are often confused.
Try drinking a glass of water instead of eating something. Your body just might need hydrating instead of a snack.

When the body gets all the water it needs to function efficiently, its fluids are perfectly balanced. Glands, nerves, and bowels begin to function efficiently. Skin begins to glow, water retention subsides, weight normalizes, endurance increases, concentration improves, and on . . . and on . . . and on!

P.S. Chlorine isn't good for your body, but it kills the stuff that gets into your water supply that can make you sick. Chlorine is normally a gas, so if you put a one-gallon, open container full of tap water in your refrigerator before you go to bed, the chlorine will dissipate, and your fresh water (without chlorine) will be waiting for you in the morning.

P.P.S. Most people are deficient in trace minerals because they aren't eating enough fresh vegetables (five to seven baseball-size servings daily). Add an ounce of a trace mineral supplement to your daily water to fill the gap in your diet.

Take Action

How many ounces of water should I be drinking each day to stay hydrated?

Weight divided by 2 = number of ounces each day

Do I have symptoms of dehydration?	Yes	No
Do I want to have a polluted body?	Yes	No
Am I willing to start drinking more water?	Yes	No
Will I drink water instead of other drinks?	Yes	No
Am I going to start taking better care of my health?	Yes	No
Do I want to help prevent wrinkles and declining health?	Yes	No

*Drinking purified water is essential to good health.

Lesson 2

pH Homeostasis: The Acid/Alkaline Balancing Act

Many doctors, herbalists, and nutritionists believe that many of the diseases raging through our modern society may have a common cause: pH imbalances, also known as acidosis.

You can change the way things are by changing the things you do

---

☑ The body strives to maintain a balanced, acid-alkaline (or acid-base) ratio, often referred to as pH, of 7.3. It maintains that balance by adjusting positively charged ions (acid-forming) and negatively charged ions (alkaline-forming) in all of its fluids and tissue.

The impact of even a minor change in alkalinity or acidity has a profound effect on the body.

It's a Balancing Act, with Your Health and Well-Being at Stake

The source from which the body draws to adjust the pH balance between acid and alkaline is diet—the meat, vegetables, fruits, and grains people consume in every meal.

The body continually strives to balance pH by adding or removing alkaline- or acid-forming ions using nutrients, typically minerals, contained in the food that has been consumed.

Understanding pH

pH (potential of hydrogen) is a measure of the acidity or alkalinity of a solution. It is measured on a scale of 0 to 14; the lower the pH, the more acidic the solution; the higher the pH, the more alkaline (or base) the solution. When a solution is neither acid nor alkaline, it has a pH level of 7, which is neutral.

The Most Abundant Compound in the Human Body Is Water.
Making up approximately 60 percent of the body's composition, water is the fluid into which the body mixes the appropriate ionic agents that adjust and maintain pH. Saliva and/or urine are ready sources for measuring the pH of the body for testing purposes.

What Causes an Acidic Condition (Acidosis)?
The reason acidosis is more common in our society is due, in great part, to a diet that is too high in acid-producing animal products like meat, eggs, and dairy, and too low in alkaline-producing foods like fresh, ripe vegetables and fruit.

Also, processed foods like white flour and sugar; beverages like coffee and soft drinks; prescriptive and OTC drugs; and artificial chemical sweeteners, which are extremely acid forming, are contributing factors to the prevalence of acidosis.

Most often, people who suffer from unbalanced pH are too acidic.
The acidic condition forces the body to borrow minerals, including calcium, sodium, potassium, and magnesium, from vital organs, teeth, and bones to buffer (neutralize) the acid and safely restore pH balance to the internal terrain of the body.

This "borrowing" is the body's safety mechanism it uses in emergency situations to maintain acid/alkaline balance that, if prolonged, has dire circumstances.

Balancing pH works like a train.
As the internal biological terrain becomes acidic (the pH level drops), the body pulls calcium and/or other buffering minerals from different parts of the body to buffer the acidity of the fluids, cells, and the blood.

The body can suffer severe and prolonged damage due to high acidity. The condition may go undetected for years.

The earliest warning signs of an acidic biological terrain are calcium deposits.
They are often indications that the levels of trace and macro mineral cofactors, responsible for maintaining the serum levels calcium in the bloodstream or interstitial fluids, are insufficient to maintain the suspension.

This deficiency in trace minerals forces the calcium to "fall out" of suspension to accumulate on bone or in various organs. Calcium deposits come from the structural calcium of blood, fluids, bones, and teeth and never from the calcium in the water or diet.

Conversely, when the availability of calcium in the blood is below the levels needed to buffer acidity, the body will actively pull calcium from bones and teeth in an attempt to balance pH.

☑ Addressing diet, stress, and exercise, along with taking specific nutritional supplements, are important steps you need to take to correct an acid/alkaline imbalance in the body.

An Acid/Alkaline Imbalance May Create Many Health Challenges

A healthy body maintains adequate alkaline reserves to meet emergency demands. When excess acids must be neutralized, the alkaline reserves can become depleted, leaving the body in a weakened condition.

An acidic body, which is common today, weakens all of the body's systems. It gives rise to an internal environment conducive to disease, as opposed to a pH-balanced environment, which allows normal body function necessary for the body to resist disease.

Acid/alkaline balance helps maintain oxygen level in the biological terrain.

Acidity reduces the oxygen-carrying capacity of blood, leaving you tired and fatigued. Also, the reduced oxygen levels allow fungi, mold, parasites, bad bacteria, and viruses to flourish and gain a hold throughout the body.

If you have a candida yeast infection, you will likely have bad bacteria, fungi, and parasites, because they all flourish in the same oxygen-poor terrain. It is interesting to note that you often won't have just some of these invaders.

A nineteenth-century scientific and philosophical debate is the foundation for modern medicine. On one side of the debate was French microbiologist Antoine Bechamp. On the other side was French microbiologist Louis Pasteur.

Louis Pasteur Versus Antoine Bechamp—A Historical Perspective

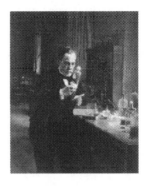 Louis Pasteur, father of the germ theory of disease (also known as monomorphism), hypothesized that germs are the cause of disease.

Pasteur's theory of disease described unchangeable microbes as the primary cause of disease. He speculated that a microorganism is static and unchangeable. He theorized that different microbes or bacteria that invade the body from the outside cause disease. This is the theory of monomorphism, or more simply, many germs, many diseases. Pasteur's theory gave rise to our modern methods of combating disease.

Bechamp held the view that microorganisms can go through different stages of development. He theorized that microbes change according to the environment to which they are exposed, evolving into various forms within their life cycle.

Bechamp observed a microbe, which he named microzyma, change its shape as individuals became diseased. He theorized that disease comes from this microbe inside the body. This is the theory of pleomorphism, or more simply, one germ, many diseases.

Claude Bernard, another scientist of the day, theorized that the milieu, or the internal environment, is all important to the disease process. He believed that microbes, being pleomorphic, change and evolve as a result of the environment (or terrain) to which they are exposed.

Bernard believed disease in the body is a biological process that develops based on the state of the internal biological terrain. At the core of that terrain is pH.

The concept of acid/alkaline imbalance as the cause of disease.
The theory of pleomorphism was in direct competition with Pasteur's germ theory. The pleomorphic theory of disease lost out due, in large part, to Pasteur's more dynamic personality and the limited technology of the day.

As a result, people today attempt to fight their own private chemical war against molds, yeasts, bacteria, viruses, and fungi by using antibiotics as the first line of defense.

Sadly, the immune system is becoming weaker and overtaxed. And because of the overuse of antibiotics, germs and bacteria have become more powerful and deadly.

It is interesting to note that Dr. Pasteur's dying words are reported to have been, "The germ is nothing, the inner terrain is everything."

☑ It seems that the cause of disease, and aging, may be less complex than previously thought.

A Modern Perspective

New York physician William Howard Hay published an alternative perspective to Pasteur in his book *A New Health Era* (Mount Pocono, Pa., Pocono hay-ven plan, 1933), in which he writes that all disease is caused by autotoxication (or self-poisoning) due to acidosis in the body.

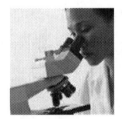

Further, Hay writes: "Now we depart from health in just the proportion to which we have allowed our alkalis to be dissipated by introduction of acid-forming food in too great amount . . . It may seem strange to say that all disease is the same thing, no matter what its myriad modes of expression, but it is verily so."

More recently, in his book *Alkalize or Die,* (Holographic Health Inc; 8th edition, December 1, 1991), Dr. Theodore A. Baroody writes essentially the same thing: "The countless names of illnesses do not really matter. What does matter is that they all come from the same root cause . . . too much tissue acid waste in the body."

In the Standard American Diet (SAD) almost 99 percent of the components of food people consume every day are highly acidic due to processing, flavor- and color-enhancing chemicals and preservatives, with only 1 percent being alkalizing minerals and natural phytochemicals.

Acid waste is excreted from the human body in the form of urine or sweat.

When level of acidity exceeds the body's ability to process the acidity, the excess wastes that are not excreted will continue circulating around the body in the blood. This acidic waste changes the pH of the blood and other bodily fluids, exerting a direct effect on tissue at the cellular level.

Also as a consequence of this situation, the cells of the human body will be deprived of their supply of oxygen and essential nutrients, rendering these cells inactive in regeneration.

That could be the explanation for why people age. Plus, with the blood vessels restricted, the function of every organ in the human body accumulating acidic waste will begin to deteriorate, causing serious illnesses in the long run.

☑ These and other findings suggest that acidic foods and acidosis is one of the leading contributors to the aging process and to various illnesses.

When does the accumulation of age-contributing acidic waste begin?

An unborn child flourishes on nutrients from his mother while in the womb. After birth, the baby's body is able to maintain the acid/alkaline balance because of the consumption of rich mother's milk.

Aging begins once a child starts to wean.
Naturally, this is due to the release of alkaline minerals from the mother. This release of alkaline minerals during pregnancy does, however, temporarily weaken the mother's body, causing cravings and increased appetite. The baby will remain alkaline while breast-feeding but will begin to reduce in alkalinity once put on acidifying commercial formula and infant cereals.

If, as this research suggests, the cause of aging lies in acidosis, the answer to longer life must lie in eliminating acidic wastes. Therefore, to neutralize acidity, alkalizing meals could be the answer. Many doctors recommend a vegetarian or low meat diet, because vegetables and certain fruit (containing alkaline minerals and phytochemicals) help neutralize acidic waste.

But, commercially grown vegetables and fruit only contain a very small amount of alkaline minerals, since these minerals have long since been depleted from the soil on which the plants grow. Large quantities of vegetables and fruit must be consumed to ingest a sufficient amount of alkalizing minerals and phytochemicals to neutralize these wastes in the body.

The body lives and dies at the cellular level.
All of the billions of cells that make up the human body are slightly alkaline and must maintain that alkalinity level in order to function and remain healthy and alive. However, their cellular activity creates acid to produce energy and to function. As each alkaline cell performs its task of respiration, it secretes metabolic wastes, and these end products of cellular metabolism are acid in nature.

The wastes of energy and function must not be allowed to build up.
An example of this is the uncomfortable, sometimes painful build up of lactic acid when you exercise. The body will go to great lengths to neutralize and detoxify these acids before they act as poisons in and around the muscle tissue and ultimately change the environment of the cell.

☑ Most people and clinical practitioners believe the immune system is the body's first line of defense. It is very important, but it has a very sophisticated partner. The proper pH balance is the first and major line of defense against sickness and disease and for promoting health and vitality.

Test Your Body's Acidity or Alkalinity with pH Strips

It is recommended that you test your pH levels to determine if your body's pH needs immediate attention. By using pH test strips (litmus paper is available at most pharmacies), you can determine your pH factor quickly and easily in the privacy of your own home. There is much to discover, so that a pH test result can be meaningful.

Urine pH
The results of urine testing indicate how well your body is assimilating minerals, especially calcium, magnesium, sodium, and potassium. These are called the "acid buffers" and your body uses them to control acid level. If acid levels are too high, the body will not be able to excrete acid. It must either store the acid in body tissues (autotoxication) or buffer it by "borrowing" minerals from the other fluids, tissue, organs, and bone to neutralize acidity.

Saliva pH
You may also want to test the pH of your saliva. The results of saliva testing indicate the activity of digestive enzymes in your body, especially the activity of the liver and stomach. This reveals the flow of enzymes running through your body and shows their effect on all the body systems.

Some people will have acidic pH readings from both urine and saliva. This is referred to as "double acid."

Your body is only able to assimilate minerals and nutrients properly when its pH is balanced.
It is possible for you to be eating and supplementing with healthy nutrients and yet be unable to absorb or use them. If you are not getting the results you expected from your nutritional program, look for an acid/alkaline imbalance. Even the right dietary supplement program may not work if your body is struggling with acidosis.

A state of acidosis is simply the lack of oxygen and available calcium and buffering minerals, which the body uses to maintain its alkaline balance.

Mild acidosis can cause such problems as:

- Cardiovascular damage
- Constriction of blood vessels and the reduction of oxygen
- Weight gain, obesity, and diabetes
- Bladder and kidney conditions, including kidney stones
- Immune deficiency
- Acceleration of free-radical damage
- Premature aging
- Osteoporosis, weak and brittle bones, hip fractures, and bone spurs
- Joint pain, aching muscles, and lactic acid buildup
- Low energy and chronic fatigue

☑ The biggest problem scientists have found is, over time, prolonged acidic pH depletes calcium from the organs, teeth, and bones of the human body.

The *American Journal of Clinical Nutrition* published a recent study conducted at the University of California, San Francisco. The study shows that the participants who have chronic acidosis are at greater risk for bone loss than those who have normal pH levels.

(J. Nutr. February 1, 2008, vol.138 no.2, 419S-422S)

The scientists who carried out this experiment believe that many of the hip fractures prevalent among middle-aged women are connected to acidity and directly related to a diet rich in animal foods and low in vegetables.

Calcium makes up 1.6 percent of our body weight. It is literally the glue that holds the human body together. Calcium is so biochemically active that it has been likened to an octopus. A calcium ion can hold onto seven other molecules while it grabs onto one molecule of water. No other ion can do this. And it is the right size to easily get in and out of the human cell. As it does this, it takes a chain of nutrients into the cell and then leaves to get more nutrients.

A compound called mono-ortho-calcium phosphate is the chemical buffer for the blood. This buffer maintains the alkaline level (or the lack of acidity) in your blood. If the acidity level of your blood changes enough, you die immediately. But, to supply enough calcium for buffering, the body must have enough calcium absorbed from the diet, or it will simply rob the needed calcium from the bones and teeth.

The more acidic the body, the less oxygen is available. The biological terrain also becomes more anaerobic, meaning lacking oxygen. Without adequate oxygenation, unfriendly bacteria, viruses, molds, and fungi can live and prosper. And, cells cannot carry on their life-giving functions in an efficient manner, because our biological chemical reactions need oxygen.

☑ The body borrows calcium from organs, teeth, and bones to balance pH.

If asked, What is killing us? The answer might be acidosis.

It has been demonstrated that an acidic, anaerobic body environment encourages the breeding of fungus, mold, bacteria, and viruses.

Question: If the door to a freezer was sealed and the freezer was then unplugged, what would be present when the door was opened after two weeks?

Answer: Mold, bacteria, and microscopic organisms that are growing and multiplying.

From where did all those "critters" come?
They did not sneak in; remember, the door was sealed.

The answer is . . . they were always there.
Simply, the environment changed. The freezer's internal environment, in which these critters live, became a more inviting, healthy-for-them-environment to live and flourish.

That shift can be likened to the shift in our biological terrain from a healthy oxygenated (aerobic), pH-balanced environment to an unhealthy, low oxygen (anaerobic), acidic environment.

☑ What is healthy for the body is unhealthy for the body's attackers.

What is healthy for the body's attackers is unhealthy for the body.

Conclusion

The body is very sensitive to pH levels; therefore, strong mechanisms maintain pH balance. Conditions outside the acceptable range of pH give rise to an internal environment conducive to disease, as opposed to a pH-balanced environment that allows normal body function necessary to resist disease. When excess acids must be neutralized, our alkaline reserves are depleted, leaving the body in a weakened condition. *Note:* The pH of the body's fluids and tissues is entirely different than stomach acid or the pH of the stomach. This focused on the pH of the body.

☑ Many experts agree a balanced pH—achieved through diet, lifestyle choices, exercise, rest, and when necessary, the judicious uses of dietary supplements—is a vital key to promoting and maintaining radiant health.

Some Common Diseases and Their Relationship to Acidity

Cancer
While the normal cells of the human body degenerate and acidic wastes accumulate, cells may undergo a genetic transformation that allows them to keep propagating to survive in such acidic surroundings.

There have been two theories on the basic causes of cancer. One is the oxygen deficiency theory by a German biochemist, Dr. Otto Warburg. Dr. Warburg discovered that if oxygen is removed from a healthy cell, the cell starts to turn cancerous. Dr. Warburg won the Nobel Prize in Physiology or Medicine in 1931 by proving this theory through his many experiments.

The other is the theory of acidic cells by a Japanese doctor, Dr. Airashi. Dr. Airashi showed that cells that survive in acidic environments eventually develop cancerous characteristics. Even though cancer cells are eliminated surgically, they recur because the acidic biologic terrain still remains after the surgery.

Obesity

The human body is very intelligent. As it becomes more and more acidic, the body starts to set up defense mechanisms to keep the damaging acid from entering vital organs. It is commonly known that acid is stored in fat cells. If the acid does come into contact with an organ, the acid has a chance to eat holes in the tissue.

As a defense mechanism, the body produces fat to protect itself from acidity. Those fat cells and cellulite deposits may actually be packing up the acid and trying to keep it a safe distance from organs, tissues, and cells. The fat may be saving the vital organs from damage. Many people have found that a return to a healthy inner biological terrain helps them lose excess fat.

Diabetes

Doctors report that symptoms of diabetes appear mainly in people over forty, with no symptoms of diabetes in their twenties.

How do they differ from each other? In general, the quantity of accumulated acidic wastes after the age of forty is far more than in people in their twenties, especially in the pancreas. When acidic wastes accumulate in and damage the pancreas, it may affect production of insulin. Onset diabetes may develop due to lack of insulin in the body.

Hypertension

Hypertension is a common illness that occurs for three reasons.

1. Clogged capillary vessels due to physical reasons.
2. Narrowed blood vessels caused by acidic wastes, meaning pressure has to be higher to supply sufficient quantities of blood through the narrow vessels.
3. Lack of oxygen due to chemical reasons, namely solidified acidic waste in the vessels.

Hypotension

Hypotension can occur as the heart muscles deteriorate due to a lack of calcium ions caused by acidic waste.

Kidney Ailment and Kidney Stones

One of the major functions of alkaline buffers is to purify or help remove the wastes in the body. The accumulation of excessive acidic wastes in the kidneys weakens the kidneys, and inflammation and swelling of the kidneys may occur in an excessive acidic environment. In order to remain healthy, kidney cells should expel all the accumulated wastes. But if the blood becomes more acidic, wastes will cling to the walls of cells, causing solidification of acidic fluoride in the kidneys and contributing to the development of kidney stones.

Osteoporosis and Gout

Human bones function as a calcium bank for the body—a combination of calcium and phosphorus. Bones stay healthy as long as there are adequate amounts of these two substances. To neutralize excessive quantities of acidic waste, the body starts to "borrow" calcium from bone. Symptoms of calcium deficiency are evident through X-ray examinations when 30 to 40 percent of the calcium in the bone has been depleted. Gout happens when calcium accumulates in the capillary blood vessels of the hands and legs. Normally, gout occurs in toe joints, knee joints, and finger joints.

Stress and Headache

Stress produces more acidic waste, leading to acidosis. Today, most of us do not find the time to relieve mental stress. Continued long-term stress will create harmful problems like headaches, mental disorder, bad temper, unbalanced hormone excretion, and other concerns. There are two kinds of stress. One is physical stress, caused by physical activities; the other is mental stress, caused by mental fatigue. Getting a good rest can relieve stress.

Man has been using herbs for food and medicine since the dawn of time.

**Health is a journey, not a destination—
start your journey today.**

Lesson 3

Acidosis

The balance between acidity and alkalinity is essential to good health.

The Basics

Every solution is either acidic or alkaline. (Alkaline is often called "base".) These solutions can be anything from body fluids, such as stomach acid and blood, to beverages, such as wine or coffee to seawater. Acidity and alkalinity are measured in pH (potential of hydrogen). The pH scale goes from 0 to 14, with 0 the most acidic and 14 the most alkaline. The pH of stomach acid is 1, wine is 3.5, water is 7 (neutral), veneous blood is 7.35, arterial blood is 7.4, seawater is 8.5, and baking soda is 12. Ideally, our pH should stay on the alkaline side, between 7.35 and 7.45.

Foods are classified as acid forming or alkalizing depending on the effect they have on the body. An acid-forming food contributes hydrogen ions to the body, making it more acidic. An alkalizing food removes hydrogen ions from the body, making it more alkaline.

It is important to note that this classification is based on the affect foods have on the body after digestion, not on their own intrinsic acidity or alkalinity (or how they taste to us). A common misconception is that if a food tastes acidic, it has an acid-forming effect on the body. This is not necessarily true. Very often, an acidic-forming food is alkalizing. Citric fruits are a good example. People say that lemons, for example, are "too acidic"; however, they are actually alkalizing, because the minerals they leave behind after digestion help remove hydrogen ions, decreasing the acidity of the body.

Acidity and alkalinity are opposites, and one is not intrinsically better than the other. This misconception has developed because the North American diet is excessively acidic, which can result in health problems. Common acid-forming foods include processed food, junk food, and foods high in animal protein. Some common alkalizing foods are spinach, raisins, carrots, and most citrus fruits.

The Problem

This short list of acid-forming and alkalizing foods highlights the problem: North Americans eat more acid-forming foods than alkalizing foods, and unfortunately, too much acid can cause health problems. According to well-known naturopath Paavo Airola in his book *How to Get Well*, (Health Plus Pub March 1984) "Acidosis, or over-acidity in the body tissues, is one of the basic causes of disease, especially the arthritic and rheumatic diseases."

Others concur with Ariola. Michael Colgan, in *The New Nutrtition*,(Apple Tree Publishing Company (January 1996) p.64) says, "Acidosis destroys bones, because the body has to steal alkalizing minerals from them to keep the blood pH from dropping into the acid range." Dr. Mary Ruth Swope, in *Green Leaves of Barley*, (Swope Enterprises, Inc; Revised Edition, 1990) comments, "We have become too full of acid and, as a result, are experiencing a wide range of diseases that flourish in the acid medium." Dr. Yoshihide Hagiwara, in *Green Barley Essence*, (McGraw-Hill; 1 edition, (October 11, 1998) p.7) mentions that, "Should this balance [acid and alkaline] be upset, the cell metabolism suffers."

The Solution

Eat a diet that helps your body maintain the correct acidity-alkalinity balance. The ideal diet should have a natural ratio of three parts alkaline to one part acid. Others contend that while this is a good ratio for active people (exercise creates a lot of acid), less active people can handle a diet with a ratio of two parts alkaline to one part acid. The following chart provides information that shows the contribution of various food substances to the acidifying of body fluids and, ultimately, to the urine, saliva, and blood. In general, it is important to eat a diet that contains food from both sides of the chart.

People vary, but for most, the ideal diet is 75 percent alkalizing and 25 percent acidifying foods by volume.

Allergic reactions and other forms of stress tend to produce acids in the body. The presence of high acidity indicates that more of your foods should be selected from the alkalizing group.

ALKALIZING FOODS

All Herbs

Vegetables
Garlic
Asparagus
Watercress
Beets
Broccoli
Brussel sprouts
Cabbage
Carrot
Cauliflower
Celery
Chard
Chlorella
Collard greens
Cucumber
Eggplant
Kale
Kohlrabi
Lettuce
Mushrooms
Mustard greens
Dulce
Dandelions
Edible flowers
Onions
Parsnips
Peas
Peppers
Pumpkin
Rutabaga
Sea veggies
Spirluna

Sprouts
Squash
Alfalfa
Barley grass
Wheat grass
Wild greens

Oriental Vegetables
Maitake
Daikon
Dandelion root
Shitake
Kombu
Reishi
Nori
Umeboshi
Wakame
Sea veggies

Fruits
Apple
Apricot
Avocado
Cantaloupe
Cherries
Currants
Dates/figs
Grapes
Grapefruit
Lime
Honeydew melon
Nectarine
Orange
Lemon
Peach
Pear
Pineapple
All berries
Tangerine
Tomato
Tropical fruits
Watermelon

Protein
Eggs
Whey protein powder
Cottage cheese
(unpasteurized)
Chicken breast
Yogurt
(unpasteurized)

Almonds
Chestnuts
Flax seeds
Pumpkin seeds
Tempeh
(fermented)
Squash seeds
Sunflower seeds
Millet
Sprouted seeds
Nuts

Other
Apple cider
Vinegar
Bee pollen
Lecithin granules
Probiotics
Green juices
Veggie juices
Fresh fruit juice
Organic milk
(unpasteurized)
Mineral water
Water
Green tea
Herbal tea
Dandelion tea
Ginseng tea
Kombucha

Sweeteners
Stevia
Xylitol

Spices/Seasonings
Cinnamon
Curry
Ginger
Chili pepper
Sea Salt
Miso
Tamari

ACID FOODS

Fats and Oils
Avocado oil
Canola oil
Corn oil
Hemp seed oil
Flax oil
Lard
Olive oil
Safflower oil
Sesame oil
Sunflower oil

Fruits
Cranberries

Grains
Rice cakes
Wheat cakes
Amaranth
Barley
Buckwheat
Corn
Oats (rolled)
Quinoi
Rice
Rye
Spelt
Kamut
Wheat
Hemp seed
Flour

Dairy
Cheese, cow
Cheese, goat
Cheese, sheep
Cheese, processed
Milk
Butter

Nuts and Butters
Cashews
Brazil nuts
Peanuts
Peanut butter
Pecans
Tahini
Walnuts

Animal Protein
Beef
Carp
Clams
Fish
Lamb
Lobster
Mussels
Oysters
Pork
Rabbit
Salmon
Shrimp
Scallops
Tuna
Turkey
Venison

Pasta (White)
Noodles
Macaroni
Spaghetti

Other
Distilled vinegar
Wheat germ
Potato

Drugs and Chemicals
Medicinal
Psychedelic
Pesticides
Herbicides

Alcohol
Beer
Spirits
Hard liquor
Wine

Beans and Legumes
Black beans
Chickpeas
Green peas
Kidney beans
Lentils
Lima beans
Pinto beans
Red beans
Soybeans
Soy milk
White beans
Rice milk
Almond milk

FOOD COMBINING
Eat to support digestive chemistry

Fruits
Best eaten alone during the day. Avoid as a bedtime snack.

Melons
Best eaten alone. Do not combine with other foods.

Vegetables, Leafy Greens, Sprouts
Combine well with most foods.

Protein
Best combined with vegetables and green salads. Do not mix with sugars and starches.

Starches
Best when combined with vegetables and green salads. Do not mix with protein and fruit.

Take Action

Am I willing to be self-disciplined in order to feel better?	Yes	No
Am I appreciative of the body God has created and willing to take better care of it?	Yes	No
Do I want to prevent sickness and disease in my body?	Yes	No
Do I understand that I have the choice of what I eat every day?	Yes	No
Can I start by eliminating the white foods that are making me sick?	Yes	No
Am I willing to invest in my health instead of sickness by making better choices at the grocery store and restaurant?	Yes	No
Do I want to help prevent a stay in the nursing home?	Yes	No
Am I willing to do what it takes to make those better choices?	Yes	No

*To check the pH balance of your body, pH strips can be purchased at your local health food store.

Lesson 4

Are Your Health Concerns Yeast Related?

If your answer is yes to any question, check the right hand column. When you've completed the questionnaire, add up the points you've checked. Your score will help you determine the probability that your health concerns are yeast connected. See point guide at the bottom.

	YES?	POINTS
1. Have you taken repeated or prolonged courses of antibiotics?		4
2. Have you been bothered by recurrent vaginal, prostate, urinary infections or sexual dysfunction?		3
3. Do you feel "sick all over," yet the cause hasn't been found?		2
4. Are you bothered by fatigue, low body temperature, sugar craving, hormone disturbances, including PMS and menstrual irregularities?		2
5. Are you unusually sensitive to tobacco smoke, perfumes, colognes and other chemical odors?		1
6. Are you bothered by memory or concentration problems or sometimes feel "foggy or spaced out"?		2
7. Have you taken prolonged courses of prednisone or other steroids; or have you taken birth control or Hormone Replacement for more than 3 years?		2
8. Do some foods disagree with you or trigger your symptoms?		1
9. Do you suffer with constipation, diarrhea, bloating or abdominal pain?		2
10. Does your skin itch, tingle or burn; or is it unusually dry; or are you bothered by skin rashes, blotches and/or eruptions?		2

TOTAL POINTS ▮▮▮▯

←——→

Scoring for women: If your score is 9 or more, your health concerns are probably yeast connected. If your score is 12 or more, your issues are almost certainly yeast connected.

Scoring for men: If your score is 7 or more, your health concerns are probably yeast connected. If your score is 10 or more, your issues are almost certainly yeast connected.

This information is provided for general educational purposes only. It is not intended to replace competent advice received from a knowledgeable healthcare professional. You are urged to seek healthcare advice regarding any illness.

Lesson 5

Signs and Causes of Candida Yeast

> **Can you remember what it was like to feel really good,
> to be happy, energized, and enthusiastic about the day ahead?**
>
> **You may even remember that time when you felt . . . really good.**
>
> **Perhaps you've even sought help . . .
> only to be told by your doctor that there isn't a thing wrong with you . . .
> even though you are suffering!**

. . . suffering from more than a few of the following complaints:

- A bloated abdomen and/or abdominal pain
- A slow and foggy mind
- A white coating on your tongue or inside your mouth
- Anal itching
- Chronic sinus problems
- Constant fatigue
- Feeling old and worn out
- Food cravings (especially for sugar) and food sensitivities
- Hair loss
- Headaches
- Heartburn, indigestion, and/or gas
- Herpes
- Intimate yeast infections and/or itchy skin rashes
- Mood swings, memory or concentration difficulties
- Premenstrual symptoms
- Red, itching eyes
- Sensitivity to molds, dampness, environmental pollution, cigarettes, and certain smells
- Skin fungus infections—recurrent ringworm, itchy skin, athlete's foot, jock itch, or nail problems
- Sore muscles and joints
- Urinary tract infections
- Waking up tired
- Weight loss or gain
- Worried and depressed about always feeling lousy

Does any of this sound familiar? If so, you could be struggling with chronic yeast syndrome, also known as hypersensitivity syndrome, candida-related complex, polysystemic candidiasis, chronic candida, candidiasis, or candidosis.

You are certainly not alone. More than 50 percent of the entire population is hosting colonies of candida albicans. Sixty percent of those who suffer from yeast overgrowth are women, 20 percent are men, and 20 percent are children.

C. Orion Truss, M.D., studied the issue and reports in his book *The Missing Diagnosis* (Missing Diagnosis, Incorporated; 2 edition, October 1985), "From my experiences of the past twenty-one years, this organism, Candida yeast, living in everyone, is responsible for a variety of symptoms masquerading under a number of different diagnoses when it invades and persists in the tissue."

How Does Candida Yeast Infestation Occur?

Adult humans have three to four pounds of beneficial microbes, numbering about 70 trillion individual organisms, living in the digestive system.

Candida yeast is one of the many microbes present in each of us. It produces vitamins, such as the B complex, within the body. Candida lives in the small intestine, where it competes with trillions of other intestinal microbes that inhabit the digestive tract.

When people are healthy, the internal terrain in the stomach and small intestine and the overwhelming numbers of other beneficial bacteria help keep yeast in check.

When the internal terrain of the body and/or the balance between the other bacterium that normally feed on the candida yeast is altered, an overgrowth of yeast in the intestinal tract develops rapidly, because conditions have become more favorable to their growth.

The opportunistic yeast population will grow significantly, producing a yeast infection, a fungal parasite, or candida (mold)—the contributing factor to a wide variety of unhealthy side effects and complaints.

Why does this happen? Many of the things people eat, drink, or take, and certain health-related conditions can create an environment inside the body that encourages the overgrowth of candida yeast. The possibilities are:

- Antibiotic drug use often destroys the friendly microbes that would normally have a protective, antifungal effect, which creates an imbalance that enables yeast to thrive.
- Diabetes
- Diet—especially one that is high in fermentable carbohydrate sources such as mono- or dimeric sugars (sucrose, glucose, fructose, and lactose)—plays a key role in encouraging yeast overgrowth.
- Heavy metal poisoning
- Low blood sugar
- Prescription drugs such as birth control pills, corticosteroids, and hormone replacement therapy.
- Stress
- Vitamin, mineral, and enzyme deficiencies
- Hormonal changes (puberty, sexual maturity, pregnancy, sterilization, menopause [including peri- and postmenopause])
- Hormonal fluctuations. Many factors associated with candida overgrowth are disruptive to the body's endocrine system, causing hormonal abnormalities that, in turn, can be aggravated by antibiotics and even by candida albicans itself.

Complaints Linked to Candida Overgrowth

Candida decomposes cell membranes, so its presence in large numbers is a sign that your immune system is fighting, with all its might, a losing battle to keep yeast under control. This all-out war weakens the immune system and will wreak havoc on your overall health.

During a long-term infestation, yeast changes into its fungal form, developing roots that implant themselves in the intestinal wall or other mucosal linings, such as those in the lungs, nasal passage, sinus, ears, and organs.

These roots enable the toxic by-products of fermentation and other harmful material generated by the fungus to be absorbed, which can result in an immunological reaction. This, in turn, can develop into a yeast syndrome affecting all of the body's systems.

A host of health challenges may be linked to candida yeast overgrowth:

- Acne or psoriasis
- Allergies
- Diabetes
- Digestive disorders, including weight gain, gas, bloating, colitis
- Ear infections
- Emotional upsets and depression
- Energy imbalances or insomnia

- Hormonal problems
- Hyperactivity/attention deficit disorder (ADD)
- Hypoglycemia
- Hypothyroidism
- Lung problems
- Obesity
- Pollen allergies
- Reproductive organ disorders
- Sensitivities to foods, chemicals, and/or molds
- Susceptibility to viruses, bacterial, and other infections
- Thyroid problems

Some health practitioners believe that candida overgrowth can lead to the onset of chronic illnesses such as chronic fatigue syndrome (CFS), fibromyalgia, Epstein-Barr virus, lupus, multiple sclerosis (MS), Alzheimer's, Crohn's disease, arthritis, cancer, and autism.

Four Steps for Addressing Candida Yeast

Purging this harmful and destructive yeast from your body requires patience, perseverance, and a multi-pronged approach. The following steps will set you on the road to freedom from yeast overgrowth and may dramatically change your life forever.

Step 1: Reduce Overgrowth
Step 2: Feed Yourself Well: Starve Unwanted Yeast
Step 3: Cleanse Your Colon—Restore Healthy Intestinal Flora
Step 4: Other Support: Advanced Supplementation and Digestive Enzymes

Step 1: Reduce Overgrowth of yeast currently in your system.

There are various ways to reduce yeast overgrowth.

Sometimes, changing your diet and making healthier lifestyle choices are enough to resolve mild cases of candida.

However, moderate to severe yeast infestations may require a more direct approach.* While there are several approaches, many may require course of two months or more.

*People who are seeking a systematic plan that is effective, easy to understand, and follow might consider the *NUPRO Radiant Health Plan with NUPRO Colloidal Silver.*

Those who are considering an individualized approach to become healthy, adding natural supplements to fill the gap in your diet between what you are eating and what you should be consuming to become more healthy these may be helpful:

Colloidal silver* is a well-known antimicrobial effective in killing bacteria, fungi, protozoa, and worms. It works by supplying and altering yeast with oxygen.

*NUPRO has been offering colloidal silver for more than fifteen years to literally thousands of satisfied clients.

Aloe vera* has been used for thousands of years for its many potent antifungal properties.

*Symphony Herbal Aloe Vera juice, by NUPRO, is cold-processed, whole-leaf juice, carefully produced to protect its powerful mucopolysaccharides and enzymes, specially combined with echinacea, pao d'arco, cat's claw (uncaria tomentosa), astragalus, red clover and chamomile.

Plant tannins* are found in a number of plants (black walnut, for example), as well as in certain fungus-resistant tree barks and resins. Tannins have demonstrated a powerful antifungal action in numerous studies and are available in various forms for treatment of intestinal yeast overgrowth.

*NUPRO ProPara™ is formulated with several herbs containing powerful plant tannins, specially chosen to support the body when it is confronted by yeast and other parasitic organisms.

Other Suggestions

Epsom salts baths to assist in detoxification; lots of pure water to help flush out toxins; consuming extra fiber; colon cleansing to expedite the removal of toxic waste from the body (see Step 4, below); rest to expedite healing.

Step 2: Feed Yourself Well: Starve Unwanted Yeast

While there is no universal antifungal diet that will work for everyone, certain foods are best avoided by those prone to yeast infections.

In general, all sugars (table and natural), baked goods, breads, refined flour, alcohol, vinegars, pickled vegetables, dried fruits, milk, cheeses, and mushrooms ought to be avoided . . . at least until you and your health-care provider have determined the source of your yeast overgrowth problem.

Foods to Avoid to Reduce Candida

Sugars and Sugar-Containing Foods
All yeasts feed on and derive their energy from sugar, fermenting it to produce ethanol (alcohol) as well as a more serious toxic chemical, acetaldehyde, made during the digestion process.

By reducing the amount of sugar and starches, and alcohol—which all break down into sugar in the body—in your diet, you'll be limiting the amount of sugar available to intestinal yeast. Check food labels for fructose, glucose, lactose, maltose, mannitol, sorbitol, and sucrose. Also, avoid honey, maple syrup, and molasses.

Processed Foods

Most processed and packaged foods (bottled, boxed, canned, pre-packaged, and/or processed foods) contain sugar and ought to be eliminated from your diet.

Moldy Foods/Yeast Products

Intestinal yeast overgrowth can result in the development of immune reactions to mold and yeast products, so the elimination of these products is advised:

- Wine and all alcoholic beverages
- Cheeses, buttermilk, sour cream, and sour milk products
- Condiments—vinegar and vinegar-containing foods such as mayonnaise, mustard, pickles, relishes, and soy sauce
- Dried fruits, such as apricots, dates, figs, prunes, and raisins
- Edible fungi—all types of mushrooms and truffles
- Malt products—candy, cereals, and malted-milk drinks
- Packaged fruit juices (may contain mold)

Foods to Moderate/Avoid to Reduce Candida

Sugar, tropical fruit, fruit juices (in moderation due to sugar content), milk and milk products, white flour products (including bread), grains (corn, barley, millet, quick oats, quick rice, wheat), starchy vegetables that grow underground (except onions and garlic), beans, parsnips, peas, potatoes, squashes, sweet corn, sweet potatoes, and turnips.

Food Suggestions: What Else Can I Eat?

For a few weeks, focus your eating habits on vegetables that grow above the ground, nuts and seeds, whole grains, eggs, poultry, fish, cold-pressed oils (flaxseed, olive, sesame, and sunflower), lime, lemon, and two servings of fresh apples and/or pears per day. Since breakfast is your most important meal, the perfect breakfast is an essential component of your efforts to deal with candida. The "Perfect Breakfast" recipe can be found in the recipe section of this book.

While you may not enjoy the effects of limiting certain foods forever, the hope is that by eliminating the favorite foods of yeast from your diet for three or four weeks, your symptoms will decrease, you may shed a few pounds, and you might have narrowed down the underlying causes of your candida overgrowth.

And, so you know there is light at the end of the tunnel, there are some delicious suggestions in the recipe section that will feed your body, not the yeast.

Step 3: Cleanse Your Colon: Restore the Balance of Intestinal Flora

Some candida sufferers experience a die-off, or Herxheimer reaction, as a result of antifungal treatment. The symptoms may include headaches, fatigue, flulike symptoms, and/or worsening of the symptoms already being experienced.

This die-off reaction may be caused by the rapid destruction of yeast, which can overwhelm the body with candida cells and their toxins. If waste is not eliminated rapidly during your yeast overgrowth detoxification regimen, your colon will simply reabsorb all the toxins accumulating from dead or dying yeast cells.

A colon cleanse will help expedite the removal of toxic waste from your body. This is especially important while treating a yeast overgrowth, as cell die-off can contribute additional wastes to be processed by the body. By cleansing your colon, fewer toxins will get reabsorbed into your bloodstream from the colon, easing the workload for your other major cleansing organs during this time of added bodily stress.

Probiotics: The "Friendly Microbes"*

Yeasts in the colon deplete nutrients and ferment foods, which often leads to gas, bloating, abdominal discomfort, and flatulence.

Though there are numerous types of friendly bacteria strains, Lactobacillus acidophilus is the probiotic primarily recommended to restore the balance of flora to the gut. By repopulating the colon with healthy bacteria, you will help to minimize many of the intestinal and digestive symptoms of yeast overgrowth.

Lactobacillus acidophilus helps to prevent yeast in the gastrointestinal (GI) tract and mouth. It can also help prevent and treat food allergies by decreasing the production of the antibodies, which are produced by the body as protection against foods it believes are allergens.

Nupro BeneFlora® is a synergestic nutraceutical formula to help rebuild the balance of intestinal microbes.

Step 4: Other Support: Multi-Vitamins, Minerals, and Digestive Enzymes

Because yeast overgrowth depletes the nutrients in your body, it is necessary to incorporate an easily absorbed, high-quality, wide-spectrum general supplement containing herbs, vitamins, and minerals, along with a strong digestive support supplement into your yeast overgrowth regimen.

Other specific nutritional support may be helpful:

- Minerals*—some research links yeast overgrowth with pH imbalance due to micro-mineral deficiency. *NUPRO Colloidal Minerals includes more than seventy berry-flavored, trace minerals in each ounce.*
- Enzymes*—there is a promising new theory for managing candida yeast with the enzyme cellulase.* The cell walls of candida are comprised of protein and cellulose, which present a difficult barrier for antifungals to penetrate. By using both an antifungal and a digestive enzyme containing cellulase, which is known to break down yeast cells' walls, candida albican's cell walls are destroyed, enabling the antifungal to act more quickly to destroy the organism.

BeneZymes®, by NUPRO, includes cellulase in the enzyme complex that is supported by the powerful nutraceutical formula.

Yeast overgrowth is a complex and far-reaching health problem, one with no easy answers or snap solutions. To resolve your specific struggle with candida will require a commitment of both time and patience on the part of you and your health-care provider. It is necessary, therefore, to work with someone you trust and with whom you feel comfortable.

It is important to remain disciplined while not expecting overnight miracles. Eventually, your body will respond. Most people report that they experience significant improvement after making these and various other changes.

The best part of dealing directly with yeast overgrowth is that when symptoms diminish, many people report—in addition to the disappearance of their complaints—their overall health has improved dramatically, beyond what they ever imagined to be possible.

Lesson 6

Understanding the Immune System

> A Prime Directive:
> Protect and Defend the Body at All Costs

The job of the immune system is to defend the body against millions of pathogens: environment bacteria, microbes, viruses, toxins and parasites that are waiting to invade the body. The term "pathogen" is derived from the Greek, "that which produces suffering." A pathogen is a biological agent that causes disease or illness to its host.

The immune system protects the body from pathogens in three different ways:

- First it has a barrier to keep pathogens from entering the body—the skin.
- Second, if the pathogen does get into the body, the body can detect and eliminate the pathogen more quickly due to its previous experience at the innate immune system level.
- Finally, if the pathogen is able to get past the body's second line of defense, it springs into action to identify the invader and create antibodies to wipe out the invading agent with the adaptive immune system.

Your skin is an important part of the immune system.
It acts as a primary boundary between the body and the environment. The skin also secretes antibiotic substances so that most germs (bacteria, virus, and spores) that land on the skin die quickly. These substances explain why you don't wake up in the morning with a layer of mold growing on your skin.

The outer skin is approximately nine square feet in size.
It is tough and generally impermeable to the environment (air, water, heat, cold, and sun), toxins, microbes, and organisms. It also contains special cells, called Langerhans cells, that are an important early-warning component in the immune system.

The inner skin covers approximately ten thousand square feet.
Your nose, eyes, and mouth (including the intestinal tract) are obvious entry points for pathogens.

- **Tears and the lining of the inner skin** (mucus) contain an enzyme, lysozyme, that breaks down the cell wall of many germs to kill them outright.
- **Saliva** is also antibacterial.
- The nasal passage and lungs are coated in mucus. Many germs not killed immediately are trapped in the mucous linings, swallowed, and then killed by stomach acid and digestive juices.
- Likewise, the **intestines** have a similar coating that is reinforced by an army of microbes (numbering in the billions) that, in addition to supporting the conversion of food to nutrition, create antipathogenic substances from which we benefit as well.

Specialized cells called **mast cells**, lining the nasal passages, throat, lungs, and skin, are part of the innate immune system. Any pathogen attempting to gain entry to your body must first make it past these defenses.

White blood cells, created inside your bones, are part of your body's immune response. The white blood cells are probably the most important part of your immune system. The term "white blood cells" actually describe a whole collection of different cells, produced on demand, that work together to destroy germs.

The Lymph System

The lymph system is a familiar term to many people, because doctors and mothers often check for swollen lymph nodes in the neck for an indication of an infection.

Lymph nodes are just one part of a whole system that extends throughout your body in much the same way as your blood vessels. Lymph nodes contain filtering tissue and a large number of lymph cells that, when fighting infections, swell with bacteria and the cells fighting the bacteria.

Lymph, is an almost clear liquid that fills the space between cells that make up tissue. It is circulated by body and muscle motion, bathing the cells with water, oxygen, and nutrients. Blood transfers these substances to the lymph through the capillary walls; the lymph then carries it to the cells.

On the return trip, the lymph absorbs cellular waste and any pathogens that may enter the body. Small lymph vessels collect the returning liquid and move it toward larger vessels so that the fluid finally arrives at the lymph nodes for processing.

The number of cells that are created and then sacrificed, every day, in the process of protecting your body is enormous. Shortchanging your body of the essential nutrients that are required to replace this army leads to:

- Diminished immune system protection
- Diminished health
- in some cases, a confusion in purpose, where this powerful army of cells and substances turns against the body (often referred to as an autoimmune disorder)

Filling the gap between what you consume and what you should be eating with professional quality nutraceutical supplements is an essential protocol to promoting and maintaining immune system function.

Remember: *It is not what you do occasionally that will help or harm you . . . it is what you do every day.*

Take Action

Do you understand that a lifestyle change is not a diet?	Yes	No
Do you know that if you feed your body properly you will not be hungry but satisfied and feel better?	Yes	No
Do you know that a lifestyle change means you reach for an apple or other healthy food instead of chips or other empty calories that do not feed your body what it needs?	Yes	No
Do you know that you play the biggest part in your health by the choices you make every day?	Yes	No
Are you willing to make better choices?	Yes	No
Do you realize that there are healthy ways to deal with the majority of ailments, sickness, and disease?	Yes	No
Do you want to take authority and action over your well-being?	Yes	No
Do you realize that you are the one with the most to gain or the most to lose?	Yes	No

The question to ask yourself each time you reach for food is, "Will my body thank me for this later?" If the food you are choosing does not have a nutritional value for your body, think twice before you make that choice.

Lesson 7

Are You Poisoning Yourself?

Toxemia: a generic term used to describe poisons in the blood.

The human body is a self-defending, self-repairing, self-replicating vessel, combusting oxygen and glucose for energy, disposing of the wastes of combustion, constantly rebuilding tissue, replacing worn-out, dead cells with new, fresh ones—a project on a scale of 300 billion cells each and every night of your life. Virtually every cell in the body is replaced every seven years (estimated to be 750 trillion cells).

Some types of cells are programmed at the DNA level to be replaced more frequently. For example, scientists discovered that red blood cells are replaced every one hundred twenty days, heart cells—every two months, colon/intestinal cells—every five days, skin—every four weeks; bone structures—every year.

On one side of the coin, this ongoing process of building a new body from the food we eat and the water we drink challenges the mind. On the other side, the daunting task of breaking down, recycling and eliminating the wastes created by processing several hundred pounds of dead cells boggles the mind.

The wastes of cellular breakdown, general metabolism, and digestion are, to one degree or another, poisonous. Another word for this is toxic. If these toxins were to remain and accumulate in your body, you would suffer an agonizing death by poisoning. The body has a system to eliminate toxins before the buildup can damage cells, tissue, and organs.

> *If toxins remain and accumulate in the body, you would suffer an agonizing death by poisoning.*

The two main organs of detoxification, the liver and the kidneys, act like filters, removing toxic substances and purifying the body.

When the body is faced with an overload of toxins (toxemia), secondary organs of elimination—the large intestine, lungs, bladder, and the skin—are frequently forced into helping eliminate the extra toxins.

When the secondary organs of elimination are forced to process toxins, they may become inflamed, irritated, and weakened. The results can be skin irritations, bacterial or viral infections, asthma, sinusitis, or a whole host of other issues depending on the area involved.

When toxins are deposited instead of eliminated, another, different set of complaints arise: toxins stored in joints result in arthritis; in muscle tissues—rheumatism; skin and organs—cysts and benign tumors.

When toxins weaken the body's immune response, infesting/infecting organisms successfully invade and begin attacking the body, or worse yet, genetic alterations may occur.

In a perfect world, the liver and kidneys would keep up with their job for eighty, ninety, or even one hundred years before beginning to tire. In this ideal world, the food would, of course, be very nutritious and free of pesticide residues, the air and water would be pure, and food would not be denatured or turned into high-calorie/no nutrition junk food. In this perfect world, everyone would get moderate exercise into old age and live virtually without stress. In this utopia, doctors would have little or no work other than repairing traumatic injuries, because everyone would be healthy.

Back in reality, the less-than-ideal world of today, doctoring is a financially rewarding profession. Fast, sweet, and convenient are the dietary guidelines for the day. People eat whatever they feel like eating—whenever they feel like it.

The food is denatured, processed, fried, salted, sweetened, preserved—overburdening the liver and kidneys. Children develop the very same diseases as their parents; because they put their feet under the same dining table as their parents, their diet is overburdening the organs of elimination—just like those of Mom, Dad, and Uncle Bill.

Every day, people choose to eat the food that contributes to their decline in health.

If you want a new, favorite hobby—like hanging out at the doctor's office, reading outdated magazines—do not consider changing the unconscious habit of eating the fast, sweet, and convenient food that advertisers recommend.

To change the way things are, you must first change the things you do. Experts and nutritionists finally agree, "There is a direct relationship between staying healthy and consuming seven servings of colorful vegetables and fruits each day."

A great first step is to examine the habits that contribute to declining health and lead to sickness and then begin changing them. Be honest! Some examples are: "I'm twenty pounds overweight." "I need help with regularity." "I am uncomfortable after eating." Some people even write down the different issues that are keeping them from being healthy.

Everyone will have a gap in their diet, so don't despair if you can't eat everything you need to become and stay healthy. Simply fill the gap in your diet with a well-designed nutraceutical program.

Remember, it is not what you do occasionally that damages your health, it is what you do every day. Eat whole foods, drink clean water, and use dietary supplements to sustain your healthy body.

Take Action

Do you eat the way your parents eat?	Yes	No
Are you suffering from the same types of degenerative diseases?	Yes	No
Do you know your way of eating is contributing to your problems?	Yes	No
Have you ever done an internal cleanse for your body?	Yes	No
Would you be willing to get out the bad toxins to help your body?	Yes	No
Would you enjoy feeling better and living life more abundantly?	Yes	No
Would you like to grow old and not feel old physically?	Yes	No
How much money do you spend on looking younger, like cosmetics?	$	____
If you knew you could look younger and feel younger by doing things differently and eating nutritiously would you?	Yes	No

Lesson 8

Pharmaceuticals vs. Nutraceuticals

Pharmaceuticals are a reactive approach for overcoming illness.

Nutraceuticals are a proactive approach for promoting and maintaining health. Webster defines a supplement as something that compensates for a deficiency or constitutes an addition. Prescriptions (patent medicine) and natural herbals are supplements, according to Webster's definition. It is easy to understand why people become confused with the difference. It sounds like splitting hairs when making the distinction between prescriptions and natural supplements, but they are worlds apart.

Before there was patent medicine, herbs were medicine. As a practical matter, local herbs were collected and used by people for various circumstances. While most people understood the local plants, ultimately the collection of knowledge for the use of local herbs was centralized with one person and passed on from generation to generation. On occasion, during the either inter-village, intra- or inter-tribal meetings, or walkabouts, the responsible person (shaman) became aware of other herbs, with different names that were used by other shaman. Occasionally, the herbs were unique; however, more times than not, the herbs were similar species, different by virtue of growing conditions and name. Exchanging their locally collected herbs with other shamen helped create an aura of mystery when the local shaman returned with these exotic-sounding names for herbs. The locally available herbs lost their "glamour," and the exotic herbs' mysterious names were perceived as possessing a greater benefit.

Ritual became an important part of healing. Whether it was incantation, dancing, noises, or music, ritual helped elevate the standing of the local shaman, because it was special knowledge known only by one person—the shaman. Once the elitist perception was established, the village had fully delegated the responsibility for their own well-being.

A pragmatist might believe that the addition of these "exotic" herbs and various rituals constituted the beginnings of the health-care industry.

Self-care is taking responsibility for your health. It is founded in the belief that no one has more to gain or lose than you by staying healthy. When you are threatened with the loss of one of your most important assets, your health, physicians play a critical part in recovering your asset, diagnosing symptoms, prescribing appropriate medications, and following your progress. On the other hand, your progress is the result of your body's ability to heal itself. An old adage, "It's not the bullet that kills, it's the body's inability to react to the sudden change in circumstance," sums up the body's ability. If a person is shot, the personnel in the emergency room stabilize the body and wait for healing.

Self-care is making informed decisions regarding your health. Granted, everyday living leaves little time for anything else, but an ounce of prevention is worth a pound of cure. There is no substitute for making informed decisions based on reasonable information. The growing market for natural supplements to promote and maintain health points to an ever-increasing interest in self-care. It is a choice to invest in health.

Regardless of your state of health, whether you are considering nutraceuticals or pharmaceuticals, it is important to make informed, cautious decisions. After all, no one has more to gain, or lose, than you.

"Pharmaceuticals are a reactive approach for overcoming illness.
Nutraceuticals are a proactive approach for promoting
and maintaining health."

Take Action

Does my present physician encourage me to make the necessary changes to be healthier? Yes No

Is my physician willing to work with me to get off some of the medications I am taking as I get healthier? Yes No

How much money am I spending on sick care? $ _____

Am I willing to spend money to get healthier and on health care instead of sick care? Yes No

Is my health valuable to me? Yes No

Do I recognize that without my health, my quality of life will suffer greatly? Yes No

Lesson 9

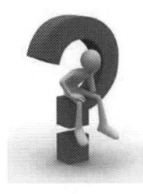

Why Are Chronic Diseases Reaching Epidemic Proportions in the United States?

Why, after years of research, spending billions upon billions of dollars, do the top five causes of death—heart disease, cancer, stroke, chronic respiratory disease, and diabetes—continue to plague America?

And why is the situation worsening?

Why are there more physicians, using more sophisticated machines, ordering more and more expensive tests and pharmaceuticals, yet, people continue to be plagued by these killers?

Why Indeed!

> To Change the Way Things Are, You Must Change the Things You Do!

There are literally millions of people who will benefit by reading and implementing this simple concept. People must understand that if they continue to do the same things they have been doing, the outcome will always be the same. Period.

Insanity is doing the same thing over and over, expecting that, somehow, something will change. You must change what you are doing to change the outcome.

Five universal opinions people cling to are absolutely wrong.

These myths are the wrong opinions that contribute to the misery of declining health.

Myth One: There is somebody who will fix me.

Truth: You, and no one else, has the most to gain by staying healthy, or to lose when you are not. The first step is to stop believing someone else can fix what you have broken.

Myth Two: There is a magic bullet that will fix anything—really fast.

Truth: Covering up a problem will only make the problem worse. Your body, given enough time and a good measure of nutrition, can right itself. Some researchers suggest that your body replaces every cell every seven years using substances that you eat. Some cells faster than others—every cell, every seven years.

Myth Three: Milk, bread, and pasta are "good eatin"!

Truth: Your grandmother was right! You are what you eat. Start eating like she did: modest amounts of meat, copious amounts of vegetables, and very few, if any, white foods—white flour (bread), white sugar, white milk (all dairy products), and starch (potatoes and white rice).

These white foods are simple carbohydrates that turn into fat if you cannot burn them (with exercise) during the two hours after you eat them.

The loudest argument is about milk and dairy products. The answer is, Cows make the stuff, and the calves stop drinking it when they start eating grass. What makes you think humans need it at all?

Bread is another one. When you mix white flour with water, it's called glue. It makes terrific paste for attaching wallpaper or making construction paper kindergarten projects. The glue doesn't go away when it's cooked. It slows bowel function and glues fecal matter to the intestinal wall.

Myth Four: You get everything you need from the food you eat.

Truth: Most people aren't even close to eating a balanced diet. And even if they were, processing, preserving, and early harvesting, to name a few, seriously affect the nutritional values of the food you eat. Stop wondering if you need supplements, and start using supplements immediately.

Myth Five: All supplements are the same.

Truth: There is a world of difference between supplements. Don't cheat yourself with low budget supplements. Buy the best you can afford, because quality supplements pay dividends.

Discarding these myths can help you understand self-care and the significant role that you, and supplements, can play in your life.

You are the person who has the most to gain if you get it right, or lose if you don't! Health is about self-care—not secrets, not magic bullets, elixirs, some fantasy, or false hope.

Taking responsibility for your most valuable asset, your health, will help you maintain your health or reclaim it when it is lost.

To change the way things are, you must change the things you do.

Remember, it is not what you do occasionally that damages your health, it is what you do every day. Eat whole foods, drink clean water, and use a nutraceutical supplement to sustain your healthy body.

Everyone will have a gap in their diet, so don't despair if you can't eat everything you need to become and stay healthy. Simply fill the gap in your diet with a well-designed nutraceutical program.

Lesson 10

Food for Thought

If I've heard it once, I've heard it a million times: insurance pays for my doctor and prescriptions, I don't know whether I can afford to take supplements. Here is a news flash—most of you aren't suffering from something that a doctor or prescription can fix!

Health is cheap. Disease is expensive.

Degenerative disease mystifies traditional health-care providers. The gradual, almost imperceptible decline from health starts when you are born, affecting joints, digestion, bowels, menopause, obesity, blood sugar, heart, arteries, and veins. It's the thief that steals life-pleasures for which we've worked so hard. Medicine may find an answer someday, but for now, there is no magic pill.

The remedy for degenerative disease is in the choices you make. Do you need to drink two liters of soda or eat super-sized fast food every day? The devil is in the immoderate choices that we make every day. We choose to eat too many processed and packaged foods that contain too much refined sugar, too much white flour. We drink too much milk and too little water. Should you do better? Can you do better? It's your life; it's your choice.

Once you've decided to make better choices, more likely than not, it will include something natural to augment your lifestyle and dietary changes. The choice of appropriate supplements is a daunting task. Unfortunately, most people march into the nearest store selling supplements to purchase several bottles of whatever the clerk recommends. Shortly thereafter, their heart, which had been full of hope, turns into a heart filled with disappointment, because the bag of pills didn't rock their world. Disregarding the consequences of this type of buying decision, the unrealistic expectations and limitations of the particular supplements collide to create another doubting Thomas.

Here are a few things that can help to avoid the pitfalls of deciding on supplements.

1. Nutraceuticals are combinations of natural ingredients, one helping the other, to help achieve particular health objectives. They're more convenient, generally safer, and more cost effective than buying

single-ingredient bottles of supplements. More often than not, a well-crafted nutraceutical supplement replaces several bottles of less-efficient, single-ingredient supplements.

2. Change takes time. Expect changes during ninety days, not overnight. The rule of thumb is to invest one month of supplements to reverse the effects of each year of neglect. The art of the nutraceutical and your body's resilience affect the timetable, but nothing will happen overnight!

3. Cheaper isn't better. In the supplement industry, price is usually an indication of quality and effectiveness.

4. At the same time, remember the old adage, If it sounds too good to be true, it probably is! There are miracles, however, but they generally don't come in a bottle. You can pay too much! It will pay you dividends to be suspicious and have an open mind.

5. Natural doesn't mean safe. Mixing all sorts of supplements is as potentially hazardous as mixing all sorts of prescriptions. Crafters of nutraceuticals consider interactions in their formulations, using them to improve the nature of the formula. Enjoy the benefits of the art.

6. Listen to your body. Everyone reacts differently to supplements. In fact, people sometimes experience flulike symptoms when they begin supplements because of the positive changes that occur in the body. However, the experience shouldn't be violent. Stop the supplement if it is.

7. More isn't better. Read and follow label instructions. It is usually a good idea to begin supplementing slowly until you reach your personal comfort level.

8. Health springs from a generally strong body. Build your body and then prioritize your objectives.

You've heard it before but it bears repeating: If you take care of your body, your body will take care of you!

Take Action

Am I willing to start making the necessary changes to live in radiant health?	Yes	No
Am I serious about getting healthier?	Yes	No
Will I learn from others' mistakes and not make the same ones just because it is easier?	Yes	No
Do I realize that people are getting sicker younger and younger because of the choices we make?	Yes	No
Will I make a commitment to being a better steward of the body God has given me?	Yes	No
Am I willing to learn a new way of eating?	Yes	No
Am I willing to prevent my health from declining?	Yes	No
Does my present physician encourage me to make the necessary changes to be healthier?	Yes	No
Will I make the necessary changes to have a better quality of life?	Yes	No
Do I want to be a burden to my family, have my quality of life suffer, or lose my independence?	Yes	No

Lesson 11

A Pretty Label and More

The net nutritional effect of the standard American diet (SAD), consisting of packaged, processed, preserved, and fast food is as much toxicity as nutrition. Supermarkets are stocked with pretty packages of food that contain refined carbohydrates and chemicals that may, in many cases, be biologically disruptive.

Today, there are over fourteen thousand manmade chemicals added to the American food supply. Each time you consume the contents of a can, bag, or box, you are eating "acceptable levels" of one or more of these chemicals. And each different can, box, or bag contains acceptable levels of a different selection of chemicals. You will appreciate the implications when you count the number of different packaged foods on your plate at each meal and during the day.

Many commercially produced meats contain acceptable levels of hormones, pesticides, antibiotics, and other substances that may disrupt the immune system, the neurological system, the endocrine system, and that generally do not belong in the human body.

What Happens When You Eat the SAD?

A sampling of a typical cart of food purchases from a supermarket shows:

- Almost all foods contain acceptable levels of pesticides.
- Most foods contain refined carbohydrates.
- Most foods contain MSG (monosodium glutamate) or one of its many aliases, such as hydrolyzed whey protein, or other equally unhealthy neurotoxic additives, such as disodium inosinate, maltodextrin, and autolyzed yeast extract.
- A range of foods that contain aspartame, a neurotoxin so powerful that it has been listed by the Pentagon as an agent of chemical warfare.

Pesticides are not something you want in your body. Of the twenty-five most commonly used agricultural pesticides:

- Seventeen cause genetic damage or birth defects
- Twelve cause cancer
- Ten cause reproductive problems

- Six disrupt normal hormone function
- Five are neurotoxins, which is the most common harm shown clinically in those whose only contact with pesticides is through food consumption.

Pesticides Are Not Limited to Fruits and Vegetables
It is not only fruits and vegetables that are contaminated with pesticides. The Environmental Protection Agency (EPA) concluded in 1992 that Americans were exposed to three hundred to six hundred times the acceptable level of the toxic chemical dioxin every day in food and water. Chicken, eggs, red meat, fish, and dairy products were the most frequently contaminated foods.

Another pesticide, Dursban, was found in the urine of over 90 percent of Minnesota schoolchildren. Dursban has been a known cause of birth defects and cancer for many years, yet it is still found in at least twenty-two foods tested by the USDA.

PLUS, THERE'S MORE!

The Scoop on Refined Carbohydrates
As for refined carbohydrates (table sugar and white flour), even small amounts of these reinforce your addiction to them; refresh your candida (yeast infection); cause you to feel fatigued; stress your adrenals, pancreas, and brain; and give you nothing in return. They are the emptiest of empty calories, as Dr. Robert Atkins called them. He had a rule for determining how many refined carbs you could have in moderation: "Take a piece of paper. Take a pencil. Draw a circle on the paper. Read the answer. That's zero."

What's Wrong with Diet Soda?
Aspartame and similar chemicals that sweeten "sugarless" foods and beverages are called excitotoxins.

Adverse effects of aspartame may include brain tumors, grand mal seizures, multiple sclerosis, epilepsy, Parkinson's disease, chronic fatigue syndrome, fibromyalgia, and Alzheimer's disease, as well as other neurological disorders and illnesses. Ninety different documented symptoms have been reported in humans. The toxic effects of aspartame have been produced at amounts much less than what is in one can of diet soda.

Unfortunately, regular soda is not a good choice, either. Soda pop contains phosphoric acid. Cola is so acidic that if you leave a nail in it, the nail will be dissolved in four days. You can put a T-bone steak in a bowl of cola, and it will be gone in two days. Phosphoric acid, which has a pH of 2.8, also leaches calcium out of bones and is a major factor in the rising incidence of osteoporosis.

Do yourself a favor, drink water.

Take Action

Am I willing to eat lean hormone and antibiotic-free meat?	Yes	No
Am I willing to give up soda and replace it with purified water?	Yes	No
Am I willing to not take the easy way out and, instead, prepare better meals for myself and my family?	Yes	No
Am I addicted to sugar?	Yes	No
Am I willing to give it up for ten to fourteen days and break the addiction?	Yes	No
Do I realize I may have withdrawal symptoms?	Yes	No
Will I do what it takes to overcome this addiction?	Yes	No
Am I willing to start making different choices to save my health and quality of life?	Yes	No

Lesson 12

A Healing Crisis: a.k.a., The Herxheimer Reaction

Detoxification Cleanse: What You Can Expect During a Cleanse

What is it?

The healing crisis, or as it is formally known, the Herxheimer Reaction, is characterized by a temporary increase in discomfort during the process of a detoxification cleanse. It occurs when toxins and wastes are being released faster than the body can eliminate them. The complaints may vary from none, to mild or severe.

The more toxins there are to eliminate, the more severe the effects of the detoxification.

The reaction is an indication that the process of cleansing and detoxification is working and that your body is cleaning itself of impurities, toxins, and imbalances. Such reactions are temporary and may occur immediately, within several days, or even several weeks later.

The possible reactions are:

- **Many people experience little or no discomfort.**
- Some people feel ill (flulike complaints) during the first few days of a cleanse, because your body is dumping toxins into the bloodstream for elimination. The ill-effects usually pass within one to three days. On rare occasions, they may last several weeks.
- Sometimes, the discomfort during the healing crisis is of greater intensity than before starting the cleanse.
- Another crisis may come after you begin feeling your very best.
- Or, there may be many small crises to go through before the final crisis is experienced.
- In any case, the cleansing and purifying process is under way, and stored wastes and toxins are in a free-flowing state. The severity and duration of the healing crisis is an indication of amount of toxins and wastes stored in your body. Better out than in!

For Others, the Symptoms Vary from Mild to Not so Mild

The healing crisis may bring about experiences of past conditions. While people often forget the diseases or injuries they have had in the past, they may be reminded during the healing crisis. There are a wide variety of reactions (ranging from none to severe) that may manifest during a healing crisis, including:

- Increased joint or muscle pain
- Diarrhea
- Constipation
- Fatigue and/or its opposite, restlessness
- Cramps
- Headache
- Aches, pains
- Insomnia
- Nausea
- Vomiting
- Sinus congestion
- Fever (usually low grade)

- Chills
- Frequent urination and/or urinary tract discharges
- Change in blood pressure
- Skin eruptions, including boils, hives, and rashes
- Cold or flulike symptoms
- Strong emotions: anger, despair, sadness, fear
- Suppressed memories
- Anxiety
- Mood swings
- Phobias

Easing Your Way Through the Healing Crisis

1. Drink plenty of fresh water to flush the body of toxins from the detoxification cleanse. Some professionals recommend distilled water as the best choice. Drink three to four quarts (or liters) per day. This will help flush the toxins out of your system and speed along the detoxification.
2. A headache may indicate insufficient water intake . . . drink more water!
3. Avoid white foods, including white flour products (bread, pasta, etc.), milk, and all dairy products, sugar, and starches (white rice, potatoes).
4. Eat light meals. Chicken, turkey, vegetables, and soups are especially beneficial.
5. Avoid red meat.
6. Be kind to yourself, and get the rest you need. If you are fatigued or sleepy, your body is telling you to rest.
7. On occasion, a reduction of the dosage or temporary cessation may be required until the severity subsides.
8. Symptoms frequently disappear immediately after a good bowel movement.
9. A good massage might be helpful in speeding up the healing process and reducing the discomfort.

The benefits of a detoxified, pure body far outweigh any inconveniences you might experience during the process. Many people describe experiencing a feeling of lightness. Others are unable to describe what they experience other than to say they can't remember when they felt better.

People who choose to maintain a high level of radiant health consider a detoxification cleanse good insurance for maintaining their edge.

People who feel their edge slipping away should consider whole body cleansing their second chance at health.

Lesson 13

Getting Started

Every day, there's a story about some poor soul who has lost his most valuable asset—health—and what he is missing because it's gone, and what he would do to find it. Our purpose is to offer tools to help restore radiant health.

Many people ask, "How do I get started?" The answer is, change the things you do! You see, your choices have brought you to this place, where your body is compensating for deficiencies or failing all together.

START MAKING DIFFERENT CHOICES

1. You must stop believing someone else can fix what you have broken. You must understand it is you, and no one else, with the most to gain by staying healthy, or lose when you are not. The truth is, there ain't no magic bullets! Self-care means taking responsibility for your own health.
2. You need to know that your body, given enough time and a good measure of nutrition, can right itself. Some researchers suggest that your body replaces every cell, every seven years using the substances that you eat. It is true! Hair, skin, organs, tissues that are worn or damaged are replaced—every cell—every seven years.
3. Your grandmother was right! You are what you eat. Start eating like she did. Modest amounts of meat (especially red meat), copious amounts of vegetables, and very little or no white things—white flour (breads), white sugar, white milk (and dairy), and white starches (rice and potatoes). These white foods are simple carbohydrates that turn into fat if you cannot burn them during the two hours after you have eaten them.
4. Amend the vegetables with oils (nut, olive, seed, or other non-partially hydrogenated vegetable oils) and different types of vinegar (apple cider, malt, balsamic etc.) along with various herbs for taste. The oils are essential fatty acids (good fats that energize); the vinegar helps manage pH in the body.
5. The loudest argument is about milk and dairy products. "Cows make the stuff, and their calves stop drinking it once they start eating grass. What makes you believe that you should drink it for the rest of your life?" If you needed the stuff, your body would make it.

6. Another outcry is about bread. White flour is called gluten. White flour that isn't cooked is called glue. It makes a terrific paste for attaching wallpaper to walls or construction paper for kindergarten projects. It also slows bowel function and glues fecal matter to the intestinal wall.
7. This is the hard one: start investing in health before you lose it. And, don't cheat yourself with low budget supplements. Buy the best you can afford, because quality supplements pay dividends.
8. Don't expect results overnight. It takes one month of investing in health to compensate for one year of investing in sickness.

So, where do you start?

1. Start drinking water, one ounce for every two pounds of body weight, and two ounces for every ounce of caffeinated liquid (coffee, tea, and soda). I would stop drinking and eating anything that contains a sugar substitute (diet pop is the worst).
2. Clean out the bowels to remove the fecal matter that has been pasted to the walls of the intestine. This material is a plug that slows the movement of wastes, and it forms a barrier that restricts the absorption of nutrients (food and/or supplements). When a supplement regimen fails, it is because the ingredients in the pills do not make their way through the impacted fecal matter.
3. Next, address digestion. Take supplements that introduce microbes into the intestines to promote the conversion of food into nutrients. The essential, natural microbes have been decimated by acid-producing foods, simple carbohydrates, and prescription and agricultural antibiotics.
4. At the same time, start taking one enzyme with each meal to prepare the food for digestion and reduce the production of acid in the stomach. Restoring digestion may require up to one hundred twenty days.
5. Finally, drink colloidal minerals. They do not require digestion, and almost everyone is deficient in minerals. And, they are absolutely essential for efficient function of the body.

Once the body becomes properly hydrated and the bowels start moving at least once every day (morning and night is better, after every meal is best!), evaluate the next step. Make a list in the beginning and another once your bowels start working. Many of the health annoyances will diminish. What is left on your list is your new objective(s). Prioritize the list and pick one of the condition-specific options to help cross the next complaint off your list.

REMEMBER: HEALTH IS A JOURNEY

Lesson 14

How to Become the Master of Your Health

Introduction

The least understood concept in the United States, and the World, is "The Balanced Diet".
It's too bad, because virtually all of the recommendations emanating from the "medical experts" are predicated on the assumption that you are eating this "Balanced Diet".

When asked, most people will tell you they eat "pretty good."

The fact is they are not eating anywhere near what the body needs to stay healthy.

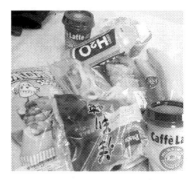

What people are consuming is a conglomeration of processed, preserved, packaged and convenience food products that, thanks to advertising, are masquerading as food.

Joel Wallach dramatizes this issue, in his controversial presentation "Dead Doctors Don't Lie", when he explains:" . . . *if you bring home bags of cans, boxes and bags of food, from the supermarket, you would be better off throwing away the contents and eating the packaging.*"

Discussion

There is a litany of health concerns that can be attributed to this blind spot regarding what people are consuming.

The difference between what you are consuming and what your body needs, to stay healthy and flourish, leads to the predictable decline in health that is plaguing adult men, women and now teens and children.

> *While the Medical community has ascribed any number of names for the symptoms afflicting their patients, most of their complaints boil down to a single diagnosis:* Hand to Mouth Disease.

The following chart may help you demystify the Balanced Diet.

Approximate Nutrient Composition of the Body with Corresponding Dietary Recommendations	Diet Related Health Challenges
• **Water: 55%+** * Recommendation: ** Drink ½ your body weight, in ounces, everyday	**Being Over Weight** **Obesity**
• **Protein: 20%** * Recommendation: Lean Meat (beef, turkey, chicken) 1-3 servings/week; Fish: 2-4 servings/week; Vegetables: unlimited (5 servings/day minimum); Fruit: 1-4 servings/day; Bean, Peas, Lentils: 1-3 servings/day	**Indigestion** **Auto-toxification** **Declining Health** **Frequent Illness**
• **Fat: 15%** * Recommendation: Oils, nuts, seeds: 1-9 servings/day **	**Arthritis** **Premature Aging**
• **Minerals: 5%** * Plants are the source for all of the minerals on which the body depends. Your diet dictates the rate at which minerals are replenished. **	**Acidosis** **Menopause** **Andropause**
• **Carbohydrates: 2%** * Recommendation: Whole Grain: 4-11 servings/day ** • **Vitamins: less than 1%** *	**Allergies**

*Source: Nutrition Almanac, Nutrition Search, Inc, McGraw-Hill, p.109
**Source: University of Michigan Integrative Medicine Dept.

There are two questions that are likely crossing your mind right now:

1. *Who has the time?*
   Between commuting, work, the kids, most people's hectic schedules leave barely enough time to sleep, let alone time to prepare 3 meals everyday.
2. *How can anyone afford it?*
   Grocery bills are sky high the way it is. Adding all that organic, fresh food could send us to the poor house.

> These arguments may seem real, now, but they're really false dilemmas—***there is one inescapable fact: if you aren't feeding your body the nutrition it needs, your body is decomposing and your health is declining.***

Situation

Your body has a big job.

- Every day the body replaces millions of cells that, through a process called Apoptosis, are preprogrammed to die
- In the course of a day, millions of other cells are damaged by the rigors of everyday life
- More cells—due to normal wear and tear, brought on by work
- More cells—due to excessive wear and tear, brought on by our penchant for strenuous exercise and recreation
- . . . well, you get the picture.

But, your body is challenged.
Is there enough nutrition, consumed in your diet, to support the repair of damaged tissue and replacement of all the dead and dying cells—everyday?

- **If there is sufficient nutrition—your body produces perfect cells.**
- **If not**—the cells and tissue, are produced and repaired imperfectly—**you're body is decomposing and you are becoming less healthy.**

This almost imperceptible **decline in the quality of the cells of your body is directly attributable to declining health**, and it will culminate in an unhealthy state.

> ***This decline, in your health, occurs in stages, over time.***
> ***It is*** predictable, but not inevitable.

Impact

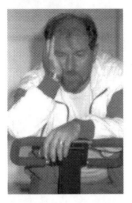

Caring for the needs of your body may be the most important task you have, because all those other things that you have prioritized above treating your body kindly, won't matter once you have lost your health.

Amazing as it may seem, most adults, teens and children in this land of plenty are malnourished. Certainly, they're not starving, but they are lacking the basic nutrition their bodies require to function and flourish.

It catches up with you—sooner or later.
The decline will start with nagging inconveniences such as: diminished energy, indigestion, food sensitivity, weight gain, irritability; escalating to some sort of "managed condition", using drug store preparations and/or one, or more, prescriptions: culminating in the miserable state of declining health.

> *You can invest in your health or pay*
> *dearly when you are not healthy.*

Solution

The situation isn't as bleak as it appears.

There are steps everyone can take to avoid the predictable outcome:

- **You know what to do . . . eat more healthfully . . . so, do the best you can.**
  *There is one thing to remember . . . if you don't buy it, you can't eat it.
- **Once you've done your best, fill the gaps in your diet with supplements**.
  Those gaps will likely be consuming enough raw, mineral rich, vegetables and fruit.
  The supplements you should consider are: **Trace minerals, Enzymes and Phytonutrients** from Vegetables, Fruits, Berries and Grasses.

These 1ˢᵗ steps will address diet/health issues going forward, but there are residual nutritional deficiencies from past years.

1. **Choose supplements** that will support the body's ability to restore that particular function..

2. **Don't be surprised!**
   The body will establish its priorities, and they may be different than your priorities. The good news is: your body is beginning to restore itself thanks to your decision to treat it kindly.
3. **Be patient!**
   The healing process is fairly predictable, too. It takes about 1 month of treating your body respectfully for each year you have spent neglecting it.

Conclusion

No one is going to get out of this life alive.

While the statistics are changing, most reputable sources proudly proclaim that life expectancy is longer now than at any other time in history.

> **It's true!** You can expect to live longer than your grandparents.

But, At What Cost?

One of the fastest growing industries in the Industrialized World is managed health care.

That's right—managing people's declining health is big business!

Dealing with:

- Nagging complaints using non-prescription medications
- Managing the symptoms of declining health with Doctors, specialists and prescriptions
- Housing and caring for the infirm, once the other treatments become ineffectual

. . . IS BIG BUSINESS. **And, it's growing**.

At each phase, along this predictable journey, there are:

- **Ethical companies**, producing aids to ease the suffering
- **Caring, highly trained people**, offering aid and comfort, working to stabilize the stages of declining health.

What's Missing?

Too many people believe that "showing up" is enough; that technology and expertise will win the day.

> ### Knowingly or unknowingly, people think they do not need to be part of the effort.

Here's the travesty: the person, who is beneficiary of the effort, often continues to practice the same dietary and lifestyle choices that delivered him or her to this predicament.

As of this writing, instances of lung cancer are decreasing in the general population.
The report rightly attributes the change to a person's choice to stop smoking. After all of the suffering, effort and expense, lung cancer is succumbing to a lifestyle change—the decision to stop smoking.

Why? Because people started "getting it".
People stopped smoking. That choice changes the predictable outcome: smoking increased instances of Lung Cancer. People became part of the "*cure*" by making a different lifestyle choice.

> ### You can change the way things are by changing the things you do.

Another predictable outcome is: malnutrition increases the instances of declining health.

It's your choice . . . just remember, you will be the one wrestling with the consequences.

Lesson 15

Slow, Stop, and Reverse Aging

Antioxidants have been receiving a great deal of notoriety lately—and for good reason. Antioxidants help *slow, stop, and even reverse premature aging* of your body, tissue, and vital organs. Antioxidant levels of fruits, vegetables, and whole food are measured using a scale called oxygen radical absorbance capacity (or ORAC).

Studies show the body needs three thousand to five thousand ORAC units every day to get meaningful protection. USDA scientists at Tufts University report that the average American consumes twelve hundred to fifteen hundred ORAC units per day, more than a 33 percent shortfall!

Research at the Harvard School of Public Health shows that the more fruits and vegetables you eat, the less likely you are to develop a chronic disease. The most significant reductions in risk of illness are seen when individuals consume seven to ten servings of fruits and vegetables per day, which, coincidentally, delivers an ORAC value of about three thousand units.

> There is an inverserelationship between chronic disease and eating fruits and vegetables

The Power of Phytochemicals

Antioxidants are just a part of a family of naturally occurring plant compounds called phytochemicals ("phyto" means plant). Examples of familiar named phytochemicals are vitamin C, rutin, quercetin, and pycnogenol.

Thousands of these compounds work anonymously in the human body. Some phytochemicals may:

- Act as *antioxidants,* protecting cells, tissue, and vital organs
- *Address inflammation*
- *Protect and regenerate essential nutrients*
- *Deactivate disease, disease-causing organisms, and substances*

Eat a rainbow of vegetables and fruits is good advice, because different types of phytochemicals are produced by different colored fruits and vegetables. Some familiar examples of this phenomenon are:

- Red—urinary tract and prostate
- Orange/yellow—immunity, skin, and bone
- Green—toxicity and diseases
- Purple/blue—heart and vessels, blood pressure, inflammation, and cholesterol

Even though hundreds of independent scientific studies show that the ticket to staying healthy, vital, and youthful is to consume a rainbow of seven servings of different colored vegetables and fruits every day, most people consume at least 33 percent too few of them to experience meaningful benefit.

Choose a nutraceutical supplement that can help you fill the gap between the number of fruits and vegetables you are eating and what you should be consuming to stay healthy.

Conclusion

Sick Care Versus Health Care

> The top five causes of death are:
> Heart Disease • Cancer • Stroke • Chronic Respiratory
> Disease • Diabetes.

Sick Care

Millions of people will endure seemingly endless years of suffering before they succumb to these killers. Almost everyone who receives the bad news, the diagnosis that they have "it," will spring into action.

- They seek out the best medical attention money can buy to fight the good fight.
- When their insurance runs out, they mortgage themselves to the hilt, so they can keep on fighting.
- And, if they are lucky enough to survive the ordeal, they must have their condition managed to prevent its return, which, in and of itself, is another costly affair.

All of this suffering and expense may be preventable. (At this point, most of you will stop reading, because you think it won't happen to you. But when it does, you won't be able to say you weren't warned.)

For the rest of you . . .

To Change the Way Things Are, You Must Change the Things You Do

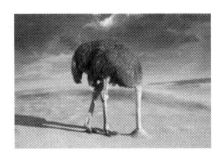

Our love affair with packaged and processed convenience food is killing us. Your body does not benefit when you consume flavor-enhancing chemicals, salt, sugar, and preservatives. When you add in the generous amount of fast food that people consume every day, it is easy to understand why there is an explosion of these chronic diseases.

The U.S. Department of Agriculture and the U.S. National Cancer Institute report Americans are failing to get the vegetable and fruit nutrition needed for optimal health.

They point out that more than 60 percent of Americans fail to reach the minimum recommendation of five servings of different-colored vegetables/fruit per day, let alone the preferred recommendation of the 9 to 13 servings per day it takes to promote optimum health.

The September 2006 issue of the *Journal of the American Dietetic Association* reports that the dietary habits of certain studied groups were especially bad.

- For boys aged fourteen to eighteen, less than 1 percent reached the five-a-day minimum target.
- For women fifty-one to seventy, the number was 17 percent.
- Other groups faired poorly, prompting researchers to comment, "A large portion of the U.S. population needs to increase their vegetable and fruit intake if the minimum recommendations are to be met."

Don't wait to close the barn door until after the horse runs away.

The formula is simple.

Poor nutrition equals poor health (with a greater likelihood you will suffer with and die from one of these chronic diseases).

Good nutrition equals good health (with a greater likelihood you can avoid these chronic diseases).

Health Care

The U.S. Centers for Disease Control and Prevention, the U.S. Food and Drug Administration, the American Heart Association, the U.S. National Cancer Institute, and most major health authorities agree that a whole-food diet is one our best weapons in the fight against chronic disease.

- Whole foods contain the powerful protector nutrients that are our best weapons in the fight against chronic disease.
- Eating a variety of vegetables and fruit helps you control your weight and your blood pressure.
- The fiber in whole-grain foods can help lower your blood cholesterol and help you feel full, which may help you manage your weight.

- Vegetables, fruits, and grains contain a number of nutrients to help reduce the risk of cancer.
- Eating nonstarchy vegetables (those that grow above the ground) of different colors and varieties can help prevent diabetes.
- Eating fish containing omega-3 fatty acids (salmon, trout, and herring) twice a week may help lower your risk of death from coronary artery disease.

The top six factors contributing to declining health are:
Poor Diet • Obesity • Constipation • Digestion • Parasites • Toxins

---

One Final Thought

In a perfect world, our food would be our medicine. You could consume everything your body needs to grow old while enjoying the benefits of good health. Our world isn't perfect, so do the best you can.

- Moderate your consumption of convenience and fast food.
- Eat more vegetables that grow aboveground and fruit for between-meal snacks.
- Drink more water (at least eight eight-ounce glasses) and less soda, coffee, and tea.
- Consider using well-crafted nutraceutical supplements to fill the gap between what you are eating and what you should be consuming to promote and maintain your health.

If you feel that your body is less than healthy, it is likely that one or more of the usual culprits could be stealing your health. Consider using a specific nutraceutical supplement to restore your well-being.

It is, after all, better to invest in health than it is to pay for sickness.

Lesson 16

Looking for the perfect breakfast?

Your grandmother was right—breakfast is the most important meal of the day.

Besides fueling your body, the perfect breakfast helps eliminate the midmorning loss of energy and supports your goals to manage cholesterol, blood sugar, and blood pressure.

Try it for ninety days. You will be pleasantly surprised!

THE PERFECT BREAKFAST

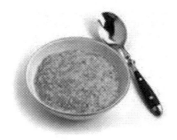

And, it will be waiting for you when you wake up!

Ingredients

1. 1 cup oatmeal (old fashioned or steel cut)
2. 6 walnut halves
3. Thin with applesauce or apple juice (as needed, instead of milk and sugar)
4. 1 T. flaxseed oil
5. 1 to 2 tsp. cinnamon (flavor to taste)

Instructions

1. Before bed, place oatmeal in a covered saucepan. Cover oats with water, allowing the oats to naturally soften over night. Cover the pan.
2. In the morning, transfer the softened oats into a bowl.
3. Thin the consistency and sweeten the oats with applesauce or apple juice to taste.
4. Sprinkle cinnamon over the oats.
5. Crumble the walnut halves and sprinkle over the oats. For a change of pace, choose sliced almonds.

It is best if you eat your perfect breakfast at room temperature. You can heat your perfect breakfast on the stove or in a microwave if you keep the temperature below 108° to protect the vitality in your first meal of the day.

PS: It's okay to fall off the wagon—occasionally. Just don't make it a habit.

Sound Crazy?

Here's more proof.

1. Over forty studies show that eating oatmeal may help lower cholesterol and reduce the risk of heart disease.
2. The soluble fiber in oats helps remove LDL, or "bad" cholesterol, while maintaining the good cholesterol your body needs.
3. In January 1997, the Food and Drug Administration announced that oatmeal could carry a label claiming it may reduce the risk of heart disease when combined with a low-fat diet.
4. Oatmeal can help you control your weight. The soluble fiber in oatmeal absorbs a considerable amount of water, which significantly slows your digestive process and fast sugar conversion, and it helps curb your appetite because you will feel full longer.
5. New research suggests that eating oatmeal may reduce the risk of type 2 diabetes. The American Diabetes Association recommends that people with diabetes eat grains like oats, because the soluble fiber in these foods helps control blood-glucose levels.
6. A diet that includes oatmeal may help reduce high blood pressure. The reduction is linked to the increase in soluble fiber provided by oatmeal. Oats contain more soluble fiber than whole wheat, rice, or corn.
7. Fiber and other nutrients found in oatmeal may actually reduce the risk of certain cancers.
8. Oatmeal contains a wide array of vitamins, minerals, and antioxidants, and is a reliable source of protein, complex carbohydrates, and iron.

Healthy Recipes From Taunya

Dill Salmon with Brown Rice and Salad

1 palm-size filet per person
olive oil
dill weed

Lightly coat with olive oil and sprinkle with dill weed on both sides. Bake in preheated 375 degree oven for about 7 minutes on each side.

Make brown rice as package directions. Each person: 1/2 cup.

Romaine, red and green leaf lettuce, celery, assortment of peppers, cucumbers, red onion, and top with a few sunflower seeds. Use Bragg Dressings or Organic Ville Dressings. (Olive oil mixed with your favorite herbs and/or a little of squeeze lemon or lime makes a great dressing.)

Whitefish Almondine with Wild Rice and Salad

1 cup almonds, chopped
1 palm-size filet per person
lemon juice

Dip filets in lemon juice and then coat with almonds. Bake in preheated 375 degree oven for about 7 minutes each side.

Make brown rice as package directions. Each person: 1/2 cup.

Broccoli, cauliflower, cucumbers, green onions, and zucchini, with lemon juice and olive oil.

Free-Range Baked Chicken, Baked Acorn Squash, and Salad

1 skinless, boneless, free-range chicken breast per person
2 lemons
ground pepper
salt

Clean chicken breast and get rid of any fat. Grate the rind from both lemons (save lemons for the night you have fish). Mix grated lemon rind, pepper, and salt. Rub into both sides of chicken and place in covered baking dish. Bake in oven at 350 degrees for 45-50 minutes.

One-half acorn squash for each person. Halve the squash, and clean out the seeds. Rub olive oil over the inside of squash, and season with salt and pepper. Bake until tender in 350 degree oven.

Romaine lettuce, freshly grated Parmesan cheese, and Newman's Own Creamy Caesar Dressing.

Turkey Cutlets, Fresh Green Beans, and Broccoli Slaw

1 turkey cutlet for each person
1 t. olive oil
1 6 oz. can tomato paste
1/2 cup diced zucchini squash
salt and pepper

Take turkey cutlet, and salt and pepper to taste. Grill. Take zucchini, sauté in olive oil. Add tomato paste and 1/2 can of purified water. Serve over cutlet.

Steam fresh green beans. Add a little lemon juice or freshly grated lemon rind with salt and pepper.

Broccoli slaw with Organic Ville Sun Dried Tomato and Garlic Dressing or Braggs Healthy Organic Vinaigrette.

Baked Whitefish and Fresh Spinach and Salad

4-6 whitefish filets
olive oil
8-12 oz. baby spinach, cleaned
1/4 c. organic, free-range chicken broth
1/4 t. onion powder
salt and pepper
Creole seasoning blend
1 small tomato, chopped
4 green onions, thinly sliced

Thinly coat a 9 x 13 baking dish with olive oil and add the spinach. Sprinkle spinach with salt, pepper, and onion powder. Add the chicken broth. Sprinkle filets lightly with salt and pepper and Creole seasonings. Arrange the filets over the spinach, and sprinkle with chopped tomato and sliced green onion. Cover the baking dish with foil and bake at 350 degrees for 15 minutes, covered. Uncover and cook an additional 5 minutes.

Fresh baby greens with olive oil and balsamic vinegar.

Chicken Stir-Fry

2 T. grapeseed oil
2 cloves garlic, finely minced
2 lbs. skinless, boneless, free-range chicken breasts, cut into strips
1 head of broccoli
12 mushrooms, sliced
3 carrots, peeled and julienned
1/4 lb. fresh green beans, sliced
1 head bok choy, chopped
2-3 T. soy sauce

Heat 1 tablespoon oil in a sauté pan over medium heat. Add garlic and stir. Place the chicken in the pan and cook until done. Remove from pan and set aside. Heat remaining oil in a wok over high heat. Add the vegetables and stir-fry quickly until the vegetables begin to soften. Add the chicken strips and stir well for 2-3 minutes.

Okra-homa Stir-Fry

1 lb. fresh okra pods, cut into 1/4 inch rounds
1/2 lb. skinless boneless range free chicken, cut into cubes
1/2 red bell pepper, cut into cubes
1/2 green pepper, cut into cubes
1 t. curry powder
Marinade:
1/4 c. soy sauce
1 t. minced ginger
splash of balsamic vinegar

Marinate the chicken and peppers in soy sauce, ginger, and vinegar. Use 1/2 the oil to stir-fry chicken until almost done. Set aside. Stir-fry okra in the rest of the oil until golden brown. Throw chicken and peppers in with the okra. Stir like crazy. Add 1 t. curry powder and stir. Serve over brown or multigrain rice.

Vegetable Lo Mein

2 T. grape seed oil
1 c. snow peas, halved on a diagonal
1 red bell pepper, cut into matchstick pieces
1/2 lb. assorted mushrooms, 3 or 4 of your favorite
4 scallions, thinly sliced on a diagonal
2 c. fresh bean spouts
2 inches fresh ginger root, minced or grated
4 cloves minced garlic
1 lb. lo mein noodles or whole wheat thin spaghetti, cooked to al dente and drained
1/2 c. aged tamari soy sauce
1 T. toasted sesame oil

Heat a wok or skillet over high heat. When pan is very hot, add oil and then snow peas, peppers, mushrooms, scallions, and bean sprouts. Stir-fry for 1 minute. Add the ginger and garlic and stir-fry for about 2 minutes. Add the cooked noodles and toss. Add the soy sauce and toss to coat all the noodles. Serve on a platter and garnish with a drizzle of the toasted sesame oil.

Jeanie Traub N.H.C. and Frank Lucas N.H.C.

Turkey Burgers, Fresh Asparagus Casserole, and Fresh Veggies

1 lb. ground turkey
salt and pepper to taste

Grill or broil
Top with mustard, a slice of red onion, slice of tomato, and lettuce leaf.

2 lbs. thin stalked asparagus, trimmed
2 T. fresh lemon juice
2 T. garlic-flavored olive oil
1/2 t. salt
1/2 t. pepper

Preheat oven to 350 degrees. Rinse asparagus and drain on paper towels. Arrange in ungreased casserole dish. In small bowl, combine lemon juice, olive oil, salt, and pepper. Drizzle over asparagus. Cover with foil and bake for 20-25 minutes, or until stalks are tender.

Veggies: sliced zucchini, summer squash, celery, and cucumbers.

Turkey Stew

1 T. olive oil
1 med. onion
2 skinless, boneless turkey breasts, cut into cubes
1 clove garlic, minced
1 stalk celery, sliced
2 carrots, sliced
1 c. fresh green beans
1 T. chili powder
1 t. basil
3 c. organic, free-range chicken or vegetable stock

Add the first 3 ingredients to olive oil, and sauté until turkey is done. Add rest of the ingredients, and cook until tender. Thicken with 1 T. cornstarch and 1/2 cup cold purified water. Serve over brown rice. (For busy cooks, put all ingredients in a slow cooker and cook all day.)

Vegetable Fajitas

4 multigrain tortillas
2 T. olive oil
1/2 c. of the following, sliced or diced: zucchini; onion; mushrooms; celery; green, red, and yellow peppers; spinach; and any other vegetables you like.
1 can black beans, drained
picante sauce

Heat tortillas in microwave. Sauté vegetables in olive oil until almost done, add beans and heat. Pile on tortillas and top with picante sauce.

Pinto Beans and Brown Rice

16 oz. pinto beans
purified water
1/2 c. celery, sliced
1 med. onion, diced
1 clove garlic, minced
all natural liquid aminos (I use Braggs)

Sort and soak beans overnight in purified water. Rinse and then add about 8 cups purified water, celery, onion, garlic, and 2 t. liquid aminos for seasoning. Cook about 4 hours or until beans are done. Make brown rice according to package. Could also make cornbread, but make sure you use xylitol in place of sugar, and I use unsweetened almond milk in place of regular milk.

Turkey Chili with Flaxseed Tortilla Chips

1 T. olive oil
1 lb. ground turkey
1 med. onion, diced
1 clove garlic, minced
1/2 green pepper, finely diced
2 cans chili beans, undrained
2 cans kidney beans, drained and rinsed
2 cans diced tomatoes
1 6 oz. can tomato paste
3 c. organic, free-range chicken stock
1/2 t. cumin
2 t. chili powder
salt and pepper to taste

Add first 4 ingredients. Cook until turkey is done. Add rest of ingredients and simmer for 1 hour for flavor. Serve with flaxseed tortilla chips.

Greg's Texas Salsa

1/2 large onion
3 medium tomatoes
1 carrot
1/2 mango
1 15 oz. can black beans
1 6 oz. can corn
1 10 oz. can Rotel
6 oz. chopped jalapeños
1 t. salt
1 t. pepper
1 t. minced garlic
1/2 t. chili powder

In food processer add first 4 ingredients and process. Stir in the rest of ingredients. The longer it sets the better it becomes. Serve with flaxseed tortilla chips or organic blue corn chips.

Broccoli Summer Salad

1 lg. bunch broccoli
1 med. cucumber
1 lg. tomato
1 med. red onion
1/2 c. shredded cheddar cheese
1 t. minced garlic
1/4 c. olive oil
1/4 c. wine vinegar
salt and pepper to taste

Cut broccoli into bite-size pieces, including some of the stem. Cook in boiling water 2 to 3 minutes. Drain and rinse with cold water to stop cooking. Peel and slice cucumber; cut tomato into bite-size pieces. Mix rest of ingredients together and pour over salad. Add cheese and toss to coat. Chill and serve.

Grilled Vegetable Salad

1 zucchini
1 yellow squash
2 lg. red peppers
1 medium red onion
1 sm. eggplant
6 c. baby greens
1/4 c. olive oil
1/4 c. balsamic vinegar
1/4 c. fresh basil, julienned
sea salt and freshly cracked pepper to taste

Cut the eggplant into 1-inch slices. Sprinkle with salt and let set. Slice the zucchini and yellow squash lengthwise into 1/4 inch slices. Cut red pepper and onion in 3/4-inch rings. Brush all the vegetables with olive oil, and sprinkle with sea salt and pepper. Grill squash for 5 to 6 minutes. Grill eggplant, peppers, and onions for 8 to 10 minutes. Arrange grilled veggies on top of the greens and sprinkle with the balsamic vinegar and basil.

Raspberry Two-Bean Salad

1 can green beans, rinsed and drained
1 can yellow beans, rinsed and drained
1/4 c. red onion diced
1 c. sliced black olives
1/4 c. red bell pepper, diced
1/2 c. Parmesan cheese

Dressing
1t. dijon mustard
3 T. raspberry vinegar
3 T. olive oil
1 t. sea salt

Mix all the top ingredients together. Mix dressing ingredients and toss. Serve chilled.

Taunya's Garden Salad

mixed greens
sliced radishes
spinach
chopped peppers in a variety of colors
chopped green beans
chopped onion
chopped asparagus
diced green pepper
sliced cucumbers
diced zucchini
sliced celery
diced yellow squash

Toss all together and enjoy! You can add sliced avocado, boiled eggs, chicken, or turkey. This is a great way to help get in your 6-8 servings of veggies! Olive oil with freshly squeezed lemon makes this a very healthy meal.

Juicing Recipes

The Ultimate

3 or 4 Stalks of Kale

1 Cucumber

3 Stalks of Celery

4 Asparagus

Handful of Spinach

Peppers Galore

1 Green Pepper

1 Red Pepper

1 Yellow Pepper

1/2 Cucumber

1/2 Handful Parsley

Afternoon Delight

3 or 4 Carrots

Handful of Spinach

1/2 Cucumber

1/2 Beet

3 Asparagus

Heavenly Harmony

3 Carrots

2 Stalks of Celery

1/2 Cucumber

1/2 Green Pepper

3 Asparagus

1/2 Zucchini

Zesty Zucchini

1 Zucchini

2 Stalks Celery

2 Colored Peppers (red, orange)

1 Cucumber

Sunshine Delight

2 Stalks of Celery

1 Pear

1/2 Zucchini

1 Cucumber

Garden Delight

1 Cucumber

1/2 Zucchini

3 Stalks Celery

1/2 Red Pepper

1/2 C. Cabbage

Spinach Special

Handful of Spinach

1/4 Bunch Parsley

4 Stalks of Celery

1/2 Beet

1 Cucumber

The Alkalizer

1/3 Cabbage (red or green)

3 Stalks Celery

1 Cucumber

Make your juicing interesting and add any above ground vegetables you like. Use root vegetables moderately. You can add organic apple juice to make your juice tastier. I will juice 16 oz. at a time and drink this within the first 20 minutes.

Another great way to get in your 5 to 7 vegetables a day is by making a creative salad.

I use romaine or other dark leafy lettuce and add a variety of fresh green beans, asparagus, onions, celery, colored peppers, cucumbers, radishes, green peppers, cauliflower, broccoli, spinach and any other vegetables that are available.

Incredible Shake Recipes

Put the ingredients into your blender, mix to your favorite consistency

Almond Joy
1 cup Purified Water
1 scoop chocolate Body DesignerTM
1 tsp extra virgin coconut oil (melted)
1 cup ice

Chocolate Covered Strawberries
1 cup Purified Water
1 scoop chocolate Body DesignerTM
½ cup fresh or frozen strawberries

Pina Coloda Shake
1 cup Purified Water
1 scoop vanilla Body DesignerTM
1 tsp extra virgin coconut oil (melted)
½ cup fresh or frozen pineapple

Tropical Delight
1 cup Purified Water
1 scoop vanilla Body DesignerTM
½ cup frozen or fresh tropical fruits

Banana Nut Shake
1 cup Purified Water
1 scoop vanilla Body DesignerTM
1 banana
5 Walnuts
¼ cup raw oatmeal
(you may add cinnamon and nutmeg)

Berry Extravaganza
1 cup Purified Water
1 scoop vanilla Body DesignerTM
¼ cup blueberries (fresh or frozen)
¼ cup strawberries
¼ cup blackberries

(add ½ cup of ice if using fresh berries)

Dreamsicle Shake
1 cup Orange Juice
1 scoop vanilla Body DesignerTM
1 cup ice

Pear-fectly Delicious Shake
1 cup Purified Water
1 scoop vanilla Body DesignerTM
1 peeled pear cut into pieces
1 cup ice

Strawberry Delight
1 cup Purified Water
1 scoop vanilla Body DesignerTM
8 frozen or fresh strawberries
(add ice when using fresh strawberries)

Banana Freeze
1 cup Purified Water
1 scoop vanilla Body DesignerTM
1 banana
1 cup ice

*Instead of water, substitute 8 ounces of unsweetened Almond milk for a dreamy, creamy shake.

**Add 1 oz. NUPRO Colloidal Minerals and 1 oz. Symphony Herbal Aloe to any of the shakes for an incredibly healthy shake!

Healthier Choices Guide—Getting Started

Cooking oils	Cold-pressed olive oil
	Grape seed oil for high heat
Table salt	Sea salt
Milk	Unsweetened Almond milk or rice milk
Meat	Chicken, turkey, whitefish, and salmon
Peanut butter	Almond butter
Margarine	Organic butter (can be mixed w/olive oil)
Iceberg lettuce	Romaine, kale, or green leafy lettuce
Artificial sweeteners	Xylitol or stevia
Cooked vegetables	Raw vegetables—make salads interesting
White rice	Brown rice and wild rice
Orange juice	Grape juice or apple juice
Carbonated beverages	Water—squeeze a little lemon or orange in it, or add a little 100 percent juice
Bacon and sausage	Turkey or chicken sausage
Hot beverage	Herbal teas or green tea
Coffee	Enjoy a cup of regular coffee
Canned soups	Homemade soups with lots of veggies
Potato chips and dip	Baked corn chips with salsa

Snacks	Almonds, walnuts, raisins, sunflower seeds (mix together and take as a snack)
Cereal	Oatmeal (follow the "perfect breakfast")
White bread	Multigrain, rye, or sourdough
Tortillas	Multigrain or corn
Popsicles	Diluted 100 percent juices, frozen
Fruit bowl	Cut up pieces of watermelon and strawberries, topped with frozen blueberries for a refreshing breakfast or snack.
Veggie trays	Cut up carrots, celery, broccoli, cauliflower, and any other veggies for a great way to get in your cruciferous veggies.

*Choose hormone and antibiotic-free meat.

*Wash fruits and vegetables; even organic are sprayed with pesticides when crossing state lines.

*There are two exceptions to the rule of eating fresh fruits: canned tomatoes and frozen blueberries show a higher nutritional value.

*Pinto beans and brown rice make a great meal.

*Add garlic, onions, celery, green peppers, and so on, when making soups and beans.

**Parents: be a parent and give your child what is good for them and not what TV and advertisers are telling them to eat. Cereal and milk may cause allergies, asthma, runny noses, and many other health problems. Teach them to make the right choices, and let them help in the preparation. Most Americans, including our children, are addicted to sugar and white flour products!

Special Weight Loss Section

Lesson 17

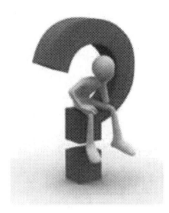

Why Am I Overweight? Who Hasn't

- Gone on a diet
- Bought exercise equipment
- Joined a gym
- Paid to join a diet club

There's always someone willing to tell you why you're too heavy, isn't there!

Can't you hear 'em right now?

- You eat too much! Just stop eating.
- Start exercising, and the pounds will melt away.
- Everyone knows someone who lost weight eating less and exercising more.

What can *you* do?

Don't start skipping meals or exercising more strenuously!
You may be making matters worse.

Start Eating, and Start thinking.
There are four reasons why otherwise healthy people are overweight:

1. Metabolism
2. Digestion
3. Prescription drugs
4. Dietary choices

Metabolism

Metabolism is the body's engine. During the day, catabolic metabolism provides the energy for all of the components of alert, waking hours' activity. The function, use, and overuse of the various components of the body during waking hours stresses and damages tissue.

During sleep, anabolic metabolism provides the energy to replace the three hundred billion cells that have worn out, as well as any tissue that has been damaged and stressed during the day.

Calories are the measurement of the energy potential of food. Fats and carbohydrates have an energy potential of nine calories per gram; protein has four. Researchers estimate that 60 to 70 percent of all calories are used for metabolism.

The body's metabolic furnace has a thermostat that regulates the use of the calories. It moves the "temperature" up and down, depending on the need for energy and the availability of calories. Also, it establishes a set point for stored energy (fat) by considering the frequency and quality of the food we eat. It controls the storage of fat, putting away energy (calories) in case of famine (periods of low calorie intake).

People with a low metabolic set point, besides being overweight, experience low energy levels and reduced alertness. Often, they are just as tired in the morning as they were the night before.

Missing meals or eating low-quality food triggers two responses: reduction in basic metabolism rate (both daytime and nighttime) and increase in fat storage.

Trying to lose weight by skipping meals and/or dieting is like creating a personal famine. It is effective because the calories are taken away faster than the body can reestablish a new set point. However, the body will ultimately establish a new, lower metabolic set point that matches the lower available calories.

When you stop starving yourself, the body perceives the "famine" has ended and begins to establish a new set point. However, because you have started eating again, you are adding calories faster than the thermostat can adjust, and you will gain weight. Worse yet, the body sometimes fails to increase the set point, which results in significant fat storage from a modest increase of calories.

Nutraceuticals are helpful in establishing or reestablishing a higher daytime metabolic set point. The benefits are controlling appetite and cravings, increasing energy, alertness, and because these herbs increase daytime metabolism, caloric demand increases, and the user experiences weight change.

Nighttime metabolism is important, too! A nighttime nutraceutical combines amino acids, the building blocks for new tissue, with herbs to establish a higher nighttime metabolic set point.

Lose Weight While You Sleep

Nighttime nutraceutical supplements address nighttime metabolism, creating an increased caloric demand to support the repair and replacement of cells and tissue, which leads to a more toned body, which, in turn, burns more calories, and the user experiences weight change.

Plus, there is a "sculpting effect" that tones and reshapes the body, and your clothes will fit better. An added benefit is the user will arise refreshed and energized in the morning. Learn more about a nighttime weight management nutraceutical supplement at the end of this section.

Digestion

Digestion, often overlooked, may cause people to be overweight. Digestion is not magic; it is a process for turning food into substances that people need to live—sugars and fats for energy and proteins to sustain the body. These very substances that sustain and benefit the body, when poorly digested, become toxins that can poison your body.

People with inefficient digestion, besides being overweight, describe themselves as pear shaped, with a distended abdomen.

They experience:

- A bloated feeling after they eat, usually accompanied with gas
- Periodic bouts of constipation and diarrhea
- Food sensitivity and heartburn

Digestion is an intricate dance between enzymes, stomach acids, and intestinal microbes—one partner preparing food for the next with one goal: optimal health. It is an orderly process.

1. Digestion begins when you chew the food. Chewing shreds the food in smaller and smaller pieces and then mixes it with saliva, which is actually an enzyme called amylase. This begins a process that liquefies the mixture of food.
2. After a resting period to allow the food to liquefy fully, the liquefied food is treated with stomach acid.
3. The prepared liquid is neutralized and delivered to an army of friendly microbes to be converted into nutritional substances, which are passed through the intestinal wall to support the body.
4. Essential ingredients for the liquefying process are food enzymes, which are contained in all of the raw, uncooked food. Processing and cooking neutralizes these essential enzymes, which sets off a chain reaction in the digestive system.

5. Shredded food is partially liquefied, more stomach acid is produced to compensate, and the higher than normal acid mixture is partially neutralized.
6. Microbial action that converts the food you eat to the nutrition to support your body and your health is diminished, because the microbes are especially sensitive to acidity (some strains of intestinal microbes may be completely destroyed).
7. The mass of undigested food moves slowly along the intestinal tract and begins to spoil. Sugars and starches ferment, fats become rancid, and proteins decay.
8. The person puffs up because fermentation fills the body with carbon dioxide. The abdomen distends when important organs swell because they are being bathed in the poisons spilling out of the rotting material in the intestines.

There are two distinct requirements to restore digestion:

1. Introduce essential enzymes that are lost when food is processed or cooked
2. Restore friendly microbial balance

Nutraceutical enzyme supplements, when taken at mealtime, provide the food enzymes essential for the liquefication of the food. Learn more about a nutraceutical enzyme supplement at our website.

An exciting breakthrough in the industry is the ability to grow and prepare friendly intestinal microbes that can be introduced into the body to help restore microbe populations lost because of agricultural residues, antibiotics, and dietary choice. Learn more about a probiotic nutraceutical supplement at our website.

Prescription Drugs

Prescription drugs may cause people to be overweight. Birth control, hormone replacement, blood pressure, heart, diabetes, and antidepressant medications often contribute to weight gain. It is important to read all of the materials and follow all of the instructions that accompany the prescription. The pharmacist provides you with a document that you must read. It describes the drug and side effects that people have experienced when taking it. The paper instructs you to notify your doctor immediately if you experience one of the side effects. Your doctor has options that may be more appropriate for your needs.

If you need a prescription drug, take it as instructed by your doctor, but don't hesitate to ask your doctor if there is a better alternative. Many times there is.

There are drugs that are usually elective, notably birth control and hormone replacement therapies (HRT).

Do not be surprised if you gain weight. Most of the prescribed drugs in these categories warn users that other people have experienced weight gain when using them. Because these drugs are generally elective, you must decide if you want to be heavy. Investigate other options.

A case in point is HRT. A long-term study of a frequently prescribed drug sponsored by the Institute of Health (a part of the Federal Drug Administration) to verify the effectiveness of this drug was discontinued because of safety concerns in mid-2002. For years, menopausal women have been prescribed this pill by their gynecologists. The warning about the side effects were there all along, but few people paid attention. This impact of this study has women clamoring for alternatives.

Alternatives for HRT have existed for quite some time. Supplement formulators have developed herbal supplements that smooth normal hormone fluctuations for women of childbearing years and help ease hormone transition during and after menopause. Learn more about a nutraceutical supplement formulated for the special needs of women at our website.

Dietary Choices

Dietary choices are huge factors to consider for controlling weight.

What you eat is as important, if not more important, than how much you eat. For example, researchers devised an experiment that caused laboratory subjects to become overweight while eating a calorie-controlled diet. Each group maintained the same exercise level and ate the same number of calories. One group of subjects was fed a "supermarket" diet of refined and processed food; the second group received a low-fat, high-fiber diet. The results of the sixty-week study were: 30 percent fat for the high-fiber, low-fat group; 51 percent fat for the supermarket group's weight.

Most people have a taste for refined carbohydrates—table sugar, milk and dairy products, and white flour and starches like white rice and potatoes—and manufacturers know it!

If you cut your portions of these foods by half, you will lose weight. And you will feel healthier, avoid energy crashes, and much more.

Packaged products contain sugar. Read the labels of packaged products on the supermarket diet. The first or second ingredient in many of the things we buy is sugar.

White flour is almost as bad. While it may be disguised as enriched or fortified flour, it is a refined carbohydrate just the same.

The trouble is these refined carbohydrates require minimum action by the digestive tract to be converted into glucose (energy for the body). When these spikes in blood sugar occur without need for the energy, the body turns much of it into fat. The drop in glucose level triggers a hunger sensation. This sugar crash is why you eat so often.

Complex carbohydrates, eaten like they are grown, help keep you less fat. Natural sugars, such as those in nontropical fruit, honey, molasses, and so on, and whole grains, require more digestive action that slows the release of the glucose. The slower, time-release aspects of complex carbohydrates provides a steady, time-released source of energy for the body.

There are other issues to consider.

- Water, for instance. People need water—period. Not coffee, not soda, not tea. Water: at least eight eight-ounce glasses every day. People confuse thirsty with hungry all of the time. If people knew the symptoms of dehydration, one of which is bloating, they could avoid many of the complaints that nag them every day.
- Fat is another issue. Low fat this and that. What people need to know is animal fat is the enemy. Oils from vegetables, olive oil for instance, contain essential fatty acids that are just what they say—essential. Nut-based oils have similar characteristics.

A common observation is that Americans are obese, and they lack the essential nutrients to keep them healthy. More times than not, people mistake obesity with overeating, when, in fact, they aren't eating enough of the right food.

When people provide the nutrition missing from their diet, it is the best weight management program.

Filling the gap between what you are eating and what you should be consuming with a quality nutraceutical supplement helps the body lose weight and gain willpower.

Lesson 18

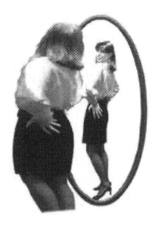

How to Lose Weight with Weight Management Supplements

People think weight management supplements are something to take while exercising vigorously, eating less food, and skipping meals to lose weight.
Nothing could be further from the truth!

What Are Weight Management Supplements?

People think weight management supplements are to be taken while exercising vigorously, eating less food, and skipping meals to lose weight.

Nothing could be further from the truth! Eating too little and skipping meals will guarantee that once you stop "dieting," even when you are taking weight management supplements, you gain back the weight, sometimes even more weight before you started the diet, because starving yourself will slow the way you burn fat.

What Weight Management Supplements Do?

Weight management supplements are dietary supplements that help individuals lose weight. It's that simple.

They can be taken to assist in controlling appetite, stop cravings, manage between-meal snacking, boost metabolism and increase energy, and to help you lose weight, burn fat, and firm and tone the body. In short, weight loss supplements help people lose weight and keep it off once it is gone.

Almost everyone is looking for a solution for weight management.

121

Who Should Take Weight Loss Supplements?

People use weight loss supplements for several reasons: reduce appetite, control cravings, increase energy, firm and tone their bodies, and, most important, to lose weight.

They are typically one of two types of people. They are either people who want to lose weight, or they are health-conscious individuals who want more energy with a more firm, toned body.

They share a simple objective: to feel good and look great. The aim is to take weight management supplements to improve the way they look and to promote and maintain overall physical health.

What Are the Side Affects?

Weight loss supplements have clear outcomes, both positive and negative. On the positive side, they provide people with exceptional weight loss results. On the negative side, weight loss supplements are formulated to increase energy and control appetite. People who use weight loss supplements in excess or fail to eat enough food can face harm or disappointment.

How to Lose Weight with Weigh Loss Supplements

Eat More Food to Lose Weight

The first rule of a successful weight loss program is eat three meals a day to lose weight. Add a between-meal snack, like a crunchy vegetable, an apple, or a pear. You should never be hungry when you are losing weight.

The first step in your successful weight loss diet program is to stop eating empty-calorie white food. These foods include white flour products (like white bread, breakfast cereals, and pasta), other processed grains (like white rice and quick oats), sugar and sweet fruits, starches from vegetables that grow underground (like potatoes, carrots, and beets), and milk and milk products.

Start eating whole grain products, like rolled oats, vegetables that grow above ground, and other whole foods that haven't been processed and preserved.

The second step is to start eating to lose weight.

Breakfast is the most commonly skipped meal, yet it is the most important. The perfect breakfast is, well, perfect. With the aid of a morning daytime weight management supplement, the perfect breakfast will feed your body everything it needs to get you to lunch—with plenty of energy and no cravings. (Recipe can be found in the recipe section.)

Eat a hearty, healthy midday meal, along with taking another daytime weight management supplement that satisfies your appetite until your evening meal.

Even though you might not be hungry, eat your evening meal as early as possible.

If you must crunch on something after dinner, try eating a baseball-sized apple, sliced and topped with a small amount of sea salt. For around-the-clock weight loss, take a nighttime weight management supplement right before going to bed.

The third step is to drink water.

First of all, it is the perfect beverage to hydrate your body. Believe it or not, the signal to drink water and the hunger signal are easily confused. If you think you are hungry, try drinking a glass of water first. You should be drinking eight eight-ounce glasses of water every day. Plus, water helps flush away the residue that is left when you are burning fat.

Become the Person You Have Only Imagined

People, both severely and moderately overweight, have shed unwanted pounds and inches with the aid of weight loss supplements. You can easily become one of the next great weight loss successes by using the combination of taking weight loss supplements, eating more healthfully, and enjoying a leisurely walk during the day.

Lesson 19

Eat Less-Exercise More Is a Trap

More and more people are concerned about their weight, and rightfully so.

Being overweight and obese are about to replace smoking as the #1 killer of Americans. Extra pounds and inches restrict activity, damage health, and shorten life; it harms self-esteem and one's social life.

The Centers for Disease Control and Prevention found that being overweight is a significant contributing factor for diabetes, high blood pressure, high cholesterol, asthma, arthritis, overall poor health, and yes, cancer.

Some years ago, nutritionists devised a theory for weight management. The theory is: the energy value of food can be measured and called calories; caloric burn is the measure of the energy required to support the body; therefore, eating fewer and/or burning more calories than required to support the body will create weight loss.

Dieting, or the "eat less-exercise more" school of weight management was born, and, indeed, people lose weight. The problem is, when people stop dieting, they regain the lost weight—and, in some cases, gain even more!

The theory has a twofold problem.

First, on average, the basal metabolic rate (resting metabolism) is responsible for 80 to 85 percent of the overall caloric burn, while exercise uses 15 to 20 percent. Dramatic increases in exercise create modest increases in caloric burn.

Second, when faced with insufficient calories to support its needs, the body simply "turns down" basal metabolism to conserve energy. When you eat less food, your body simply adapts to fewer calories. Rebound weight gain occurs after the diet is discontinued, because the caloric intake increases more quickly than lower basal metabolism that was set for consumption of fewer calories.

A solid weight management program requires moderate exercise, better nutrition, and a catalyst to promote basal metabolism. In many cases, that catalyst is a dietary supplement.

Here are examples of nutraceutical supplements that support weight loss.

The daytime supplement promotes weight loss and helps regulate appetite, metabolism, and energy. The nighttime supplement helps tone and firm the body and promotes stress management and restful sleep. Together, they offer a powerful tool to help you feel good and look great around the clock.

Choosing to lose weight is one thing—making the changes that will keep it off is the smartest, healthiest decision you will ever make.

Lesson 20

The Three-Day Diet

You can lose up to ten pounds in three days.

This three-day diet is one of the most popular ways to jump-start weight loss because it works! There are a few rules to follow for successful weight loss:

- Do not vary or substitute any of the listed foods.
- Salt and pepper may be used but no other seasonings.
- Where no quantity is given, there are no restrictions other than common sense.
- This diet is to be used three days at a time. After three days of dieting, you may eat normal food, but do not overdo it. After your four days of normal eating, start back on your three-day diet.
- Drink eight glasses of water each day.

1st Day

Breakfast: Black coffee or tea, 1/2 grapefruit, 1 slice of toast, 2 tbsp. peanut butter

Lunch: 1/2 cup tuna, 1 slice of toast, coffee or tea

Dinner: 2 slices any type of meat (about 3 oz.), 1 cup string beans, 1 cup beets, 1 small apple, 1 cup low-fat frozen yogurt

2nd Day:

Breakfast: 1 egg, 1/2 banana, 1 slice of toast, black coffee or tea

Lunch: 1 cup of cottage cheese, 5 saltine crackers

Dinner: 1 skinless chicken breast, 1 cup broccoli, 1/2 cup of carrots, 1/2 banana, 1/2 cup low-fat frozen yogurt

3rd Day:

Breakfast: 5 saltine crackers, 1 slice of cheddar cheese, 1 small apple, black coffee or tea

Lunch: 1 hard-boiled egg, 1 slice of toast

Dinner: 1 cup of tuna, 1 cup of beets, 1 cup of cauliflower, 1/2 cantaloupe, 1/2 cup low-fat frozen yogurt

NOTE: Individual weight loss may vary; be patient and stick to it. Most people will lose ten pounds.

Insanity is: doing the same thing over and over, expecting a different outcome. You must change the things you do to change the way things are.

During my healing, I spent untold hours with my Lord and Savior, Jesus Christ. I drew strength and comfort from Him. I read the Bible daily to strengthen my relationship with Him.

If you do not know Jesus, I would like to invite you to ask Him into your heart by saying the following prayer.

Heavenly Father, I thank you for sending your son, Jesus, to die on the cross for my sins.

I repent of my sins and ask that Jesus come into my heart today to be my Lord and Savior.

I ask that the Holy Spirit guide me each day into the knowledge of who I am in Christ.

Thank you for loving me and giving me a new life, a life of blessing and favor. Help me to live the life that Jesus' death on the cross allows me to live, and help me to become the person you created me to be. In Jesus' precious name, amen.

You are a precious child of the King of Kings! He loves you with an everlasting love. He gave His life for you to have peace in your heart and health in your body. Praise His name for all He has done for us! Do all you can to be all He has made you to be and love one another as He has loved us. I pray Gods' supernatural peace in your heart and that fear or worry can no longer be in your life. Shalom!

Jeanie's testimony can be read in her book, *The Healing Gift—Defeating Cancer*.

For more information and life-changing nutraceutical products, please visit our website:

www.creatingradianthealth.com

About the Authors

Frank Lucas and Jeanie Traub are internationally known Natural Health Consultants. They both have authored other books and have been helping others achieve health for numerous years.

Frank has dedicated the last 20 plus years to Interactive Medicine and the research and development of professional grade nutraceutical products. He is the president and CEO of Nupro Nutraceutical Products based in Castle Rock, Colorado, U.S.A. He has served on numerous Boards of Directors and is currently a member of the Advisory Board for a highly respected U.S. dietary supplement laboratory. Frank is also a speaker, lecturer, teacher and consultant on health and nutrition.

Jeanie has been working with Frank for the last several years. She is a speaker, teacher, consultant and an ordained minister. She has been featured on Christian television and numerous radio shows. Jeanie has dedicated her studies to specializing in nutrition for cancer patients and preventative nutrition. Through her cancer ministry Jeanie has ministered to many people through their personal battle with cancer.